# The Self-Esteem Journal

Alison Waines played the cello professionally before making a career change and qualifying as a psychotherapist and counsellor in 1995. Since then, she has worked in private practice, achieving senior accreditation status in 2008. Also a qualified teacher, Alison has designed and presented courses on self-esteem and guided meditation, together with a range of personal development workshops. She has written extensively for *Slimming World* magazine and has made live appearances on television and radio. In 2008, Alison began writing psychological thrillers and, writing as A. J. Waines, has secured publishing deals for her first two novels. She lives in Southampton with her husband.

# Overcoming Common Problems Series

*Selected titles*

A full list of titles is available from Sheldon Press,
36 Causton Street, London SW1P 4ST and on our website at
www.sheldonpress.co.uk

Overcoming Common Problems

# The Self-Esteem Journal

ALISON WAINES

**sheldon** **PRESS**

*To my parents, Mary and Gordon, for supporting me always,
every step of the way.*

*I owe much gratitude to all the clients who have enabled me to
develop journal techniques and who have enriched my learning
and development.*

*I particularly want to thank my wonderful husband Matthew,
for his encouragement and for the hours he has spent helping
me to pull the book into shape.*

First published in Great Britain in 2004

Sheldon Press
36 Causton Street
London SW1P 4ST
www.sheldonpress.co.uk

Reprinted four times
Second edition published 2013

Copyright © Alison Waines 2004, 2013

The author and publisher have made every effort to ensure that the
external website and email addresses included in this book are correct and
up to date at the time of going to press. The author and publisher are not
responsible for the content, quality or continuing accessibility of the sites.

*British Library Cataloguing-in-Publication Data*
A catalogue record for this book is available from the British Library

ISBN 978-1-84709-297-7
eBook ISBN 978-1-84709-315-8

Typeset by Fakenham Prepress Solutions, Fakenham, Norfolk NR21 8NN
Printed in Great Britain by Ashford Colour Press
Subsequently digitally printed in Great Britain

# Contents

# Introduction

## Self-esteem and keeping a journal

The most common problem I see facing clients who come to me for counselling is low self-esteem. Although people might describe their problems using terms like 'depression', 'anxiety', 'relationship breakdown', 'lack of motivation', or 'an eating disorder', more often than not a lack of self-esteem is at the source. Low self-esteem can leave people feeling inadequate and unworthy, ashamed, awkward and unable to handle some of life's difficult situations with confidence.

Keeping a journal is one of the most therapeutic tools I know for improving self-esteem. I have discovered that those men and women who have kept a 'self-esteem journal' as part of their counselling have changed their lives more quickly and more deeply than those who have sought counselling on its own. All the clients I have worked with using the journal techniques described in this book (over 300) have found them useful in building self-esteem to some degree.

I encourage most clients to start using a journal from our very first session together, whether their problems seem to involve self-esteem or not. Through keeping a journal they are learning to express their feelings in more depth and finding an alternative approach to the 'stiff upper-lip' mentality which many of us are encouraged to abide by. By writing regular private records of their feelings, thoughts and experiences, and by working through specific exercises, they open up a new and better relationship with themselves. This improved relationship with oneself is at the heart of self-esteem.

## How a journal helped me

I have kept a journal on and off ever since the age of nine. In the beginning, it served merely as a container for outpourings about pop stars, boys and the anguish of puberty. It was only much later, when I began to be aware of *how* I was using this journal, that I could see the ways it could help me more constructively. For much of my late twenties I had low self-esteem. I felt a lack of confidence and a compulsion to try to 'improve' myself. I was a wallflower at parties and felt self-conscious in social situations. Others seemed to sparkle with wit and humour, whereas I felt boring and dull. I wanted to reinvent my life. I did not seem able to value myself at that time and wanted to 'become someone else'. It was then that my journal became a lifeline; a place where I could learn to listen to myself, develop self-awareness and start to honour my feelings and ways of coping with the world. Through writing down the intricacies of my inner turmoil I began to understand myself better and as a result my self-esteem increased. I was no longer interested in being anyone else – I liked and wanted to be myself completely.

Since that time I have collected, adapted and devised many therapeutic exercises and journal techniques aimed at developing self-esteem. In recent years my journal has become a witness to my own journey of personal development, holding my dreams, dilemmas, fears and triumphs, and helping me to work through decisions about my career, relationships and lifestyle. It has been a decisive support not only in helping me to clarify who I am and what I want from life, but in helping me to put my ideas and plans into practice.

Now, my journal is always there, always ready to 'listen' to me. What's more, it costs next to nothing. This marvellous tool, which consists of a few scraps of paper and a biro, helps me to work through my difficulties and turn worries into problem-solving. It is a place where I can express and examine my unchartered inner emotional life, helping me to get to know myself inside out. On a regular basis it helps me to step off the roller-coaster of life's events and day-to-day activities to see where I am, in order to 'sort myself out'. Through the use of a journal, I have developed a new relation-ship with myself, so that I now respect and cherish who I am more consistently than before.

## About this book

This book will show you what I have learnt about self-esteem and confidence over the years, and how you might make use of these lessons for yourself. There are also examples of the turning points achieved by some of the clients in my practice. I hope their experiences and journal extracts will give you inspiration and insight into the ways in which a journal could be useful for you.

The relationship you have with yourself is at the heart of self-esteem. In a practical way, I aim to help you to improve this relationship with yourself and to enjoy *being* yourself more. Step-by-step exercises throughout the text will invite you to explore the way you feel about yourself and examine your patterns of behaviours and beliefs. Your writing in response to the exercises will help you to develop many areas of self-esteem, so that you can get to know yourself better and offer yourself more compassion, respect, acceptance and support.

The exercises are intended to enable you, through developing self-awareness and simple shifts in your attitudes and behaviours, to achieve the deep transformations necessary for creating genuine and long-lasting self-esteem. I hope they will help you to like and love yourself and build close and rewarding relationships with other people.

## Who is the self-esteem journal for?

The self-esteem journal can be used by anyone who has ever lacked self-esteem. It is for anyone who has ever felt inadequate and longed to become a 'better' or different person. The self-esteem journal is also designed for people such as counsellors and psychotherapists, who want to help others who are currently suffering from low self-esteem. It is a resource for student counsellors and established practitioners alike, offering tools and techniques to use with clients. No matter what your age, occupation or position in life, you can start using a journal to help you to discover a more fulfilling and complete way of being.

## How to use this book

The self-esteem journal is a resource book of exercises, techniques and examples to help you get started on your own journal or to help you to refresh a journal which you are already keeping. It will give you lots of different ideas for developing your self-esteem and for working towards getting the best out of your life.

The exercises offer a framework for you to explore and develop self-esteem in all areas of your life – your work, relationships, family, home life, social life, your past and your hopes for the future. It is also written to help you to deal with difficulties, such as blocks to moving forward, doubts about yourself, failings, fears, guilt, shame, confusion, emotional pain, depression, anxiety and so on.

Most of the exercises are simple and straightforward and you need no prior experience of writing a journal. You can explore the exercises in any order you wish (you could, for example, start with the 'quick journal tools' described in Chapter 12) and you do not need to read from cover to cover before you get started.

Using these techniques as a stimulus, I hope you will begin to make your own transformation towards improved self-esteem.

# 1

# How the self-esteem journal works

## How the self-esteem journal can help you

Your own self-esteem journal can be a private and confidential record of your deepest feelings and thoughts. It can be your best friend when there is no one else around to turn to, or when you are reluctant to tell someone else about your state of mind. Your journal can be a rehearsal space to bring together your thoughts and emotions before you decide to reveal information to others. It can be a great release in encouraging you to empty thoughts and feelings out of your head and to help you to make some sense of them.

### Annette, nursery nurse, 28
I cannot tell you how much keeping a journal has helped me over the past eight months. I was so busy 'doing' all the time that I hadn't realized how little I listen. Not only have I not listened to others, but most significantly I have not listened to myself. Now I give myself this space. I have found such tremendous relief and release through writing down my thoughts and feelings and I have much more respect for these parts of myself now. I have used the journal to bring me more awareness of my own inner resources and this has improved my self-esteem in so many ways.

Through keeping a self-esteem journal you can work towards:

- Developing your self-awareness and noticing any patterns you may be repeating.
- Tackling problems and finding solutions.
- Gaining a clearer sense of direction and purpose in your life.
- Understanding yourself more and why you respond in particular ways to things.
- Becoming more supportive to yourself.
- Improving your ways of relating to and dealing with other people.

5

- Starting to break habits and destructive behaviour patterns.
- Developing a record of strengths and resources which help you through bad times.
- Seeing how you are changing and moving forward.
- Recognizing important milestones.
- Discovering what works well in your life, so that you can create more of it.

All of these factors have the potential to improve your self-esteem.

## What is a journal?

The word 'journal' comes from the old Latin adjective 'diurnalis' meaning 'daily', and is also associated with the French noun 'journée', meaning 'day's work or travel'. In 1605, a reference was made by Ben Jonson to a book designed for keeping a daily record, called a 'Diary', and earlier examples recording daily personal reflections go back as far as the tenth century in Japan.

Journals and diaries (throughout this book I use the terms 'journal' and 'diary' synonymously) have been written by men and women for centuries, giving us unique insights into their public and private lives.

Many of these documents still exist today, such as the diaries of Samuel Pepys, whose records give a fascinating perspective on London's social and political history between 1660 and 1669. More recent personal diaries include those of Anaïs Nin, which detail her amorous encounters during the 1920s, and that of Anne Frank, who wrote a poignant account of her days confined in a secret annexe during the Second World War. Popular fiction diaries, such as *The Diary of Adrian Mole* (Sue Townsend) and *Bridget Jones's Diary* (Helen Fielding), allow the reader to 'eavesdrop' on the private hang-ups, trivial embarrassments and secret dreams of the characters.

## A therapeutic journal

Various kinds of journal will be discussed in this book (creating a dream journal, pillow book and mind-maps, for example). Their common theme is that they are all 'therapeutic', meaning they are aimed at *helping* the journal-writer in some way. Unlike many published journals, a therapeutic journal is not designed to be read by anyone else. It belongs to the writer alone and is a safe space for revealing innermost thoughts.

A therapeutic journal will be based on personal reflection and not merely on a record of activities, so privacy and confidentiality are of great importance. It will not be a conventional 'had lunch' kind of diary, but instead will contain outpourings of feelings, thoughts, ideas and plans about a whole range of issues in your life. In this way *you*, and not the events happening around you, will be at the centre of your journal.

## What is self-esteem?

The kind of journal-writing explored in this book is designed to help you to develop many areas of self-esteem. Essentially self-esteem is the kind of relationship you have with yourself – the ways you value yourself on a day-to-day basis. It is difficult to be fulfilled and satisfied in whatever you do if you do not feel worthwhile or good about yourself. Throughout this book, 'low self-esteem' will refer to feelings of inadequacy, lack of self-valuing and self-worth, whereas 'higher' or 'high self-esteem' will refer to feelings of worthiness, loving oneself and feeling significant.

One way in which self-esteem can be measured is by noticing how you silently 'talk to yourself' throughout the day. We all have this silent inner monologue going on continuously whenever we are awake – it might go something like this:

I must remember to get milk on the way home from work ... I wonder if Mum has phoned ... I feel a bit embarrassed about talking to this man at the bus-stop ... where's my ticket? ... I bet he's going to jump the queue ...

This kind of 'self-talk' is so automatic that we may pay very little attention to it and barely notice it is there.

People with low self-esteem tend to *put themselves down* through this inner self-talk and may not even know that they are doing it, for example:

Oh, there I go making a complete fool of myself again ... I'm so stupid ... no one's going to ask me to the Christmas party, and if they do I'll pretend I'm busy, because I'm so useless at parties ... everyone is much more entertaining than me ... I wish I was like that woman over there, she looks so confident ...

People with higher self-esteem tend *to support themselves and take care of themselves* through this inner chit-chat:

I'm feeling really nervous about work, but it's OK, it's because I'm new at this job and I can't be expected to know everything ... I might need to ask for some help and that's OK, I can do that without feeling embarrassed ... I am feeling really tired and I don't know why – so I'll make sure I get lots of sleep and take it easy over the next few days ...

The way in which you talk to yourself, on and off through the day, is an immediate indicator of how much you respect and like yourself. We will explore this self-talk in more detail in Chapters 5 and 6.

Self-esteem also embraces how well you understand, accept and forgive yourself. High self-esteem includes effective coping skills, self-confidence, assertiveness and resilience to setbacks. It usually gives you an inner security and stability, where you can trust yourself and your judgement. High self-esteem means being able to see choices, possibilities and make clear decisions for yourself. It means being able to relate and connect openly to others, to take responsibility and be accountable for the consequences of your actions. All of these areas will be explored in this book.

## Where does self-esteem come from?

We learn how to value ourselves through the ways in which others have valued us in the past. Imagine the level of self-esteem a five-year-old child is likely to have if she has been told one hundred times each day that she is naughty, difficult, a nuisance or unwanted. Compare this to the child who is told as many times that they are clever, good, loved and doing well. We tend to internalize the types of judgement we receive from parents, school, siblings and friends from an early age and my work has taught me that these judgements often stay with us to form the basis of the internal monologue we have with ourselves every day.

As children, we not only receive these external judgements from others, but we begin to make comparisons with our peers. We notice that we are taller or shorter than our schoolmates, slimmer or fatter, less good at maths or better at games. We make our own inner judgements on the basis of these comparisons and on how others respond to us. The world is like a mirror showing us where we fit in to the overall scheme of things, in terms of intelligence, personality, character, abilities and achievements.

In addition to this, all of us will have different ways of *interpreting* external circumstances and responses from others. Interpretation is the personal meaning we make of certain events or interactions, which is often influenced or 'coloured' by previous experience. This is partly due to the individual way we view and experience the world, but may also be due in part to how we were treated when we were very young. For example, a little boy whose mother was largely absent during his infant years (perhaps due to pressure to earn a living) may interpret this absence to mean that he was not valued. His interpretation was that his mother did not love him enough to want to spend time with him. Later in his life, the boy's mother may repeatedly try to explain the absence to him. She may tell him that there were other reasons for the absence; that she worked in order to support him, but it is the absence that the boy remembers and he may take the feelings and expectation of not being valued into his adult life.

Much low self-esteem starts at school, when children are often rated and ranked among others of the same age. An 'A' grade child gets positive messages from the teacher and the 'D' grade child gets negative ones. This system does not help to build self-esteem in children and adolescents. Instead it helps them to measure themselves in particular ways, to undervalue the differences, and to draw conclusions for themselves about how 'worthwhile' they are.

One client, Sylvia, realized through her journal that her low self-esteem was linked to her father's response to her achievements as a child:

**Sylvia, publishing assistant, 32**
I always remember a nagging feeling ever since I was a child of not feeling good enough. I would bring home glowing school reports and my father would pick on the one subject where I got a 'C' and

be annoyed with me. I felt like a real disappointment and developed an unrealistic sense of perfectionism, which meant I inevitably failed in everything I tried to do. After working on journal techniques I was able to turn things around. By writing regularly, I could clearly notice my habitual thought patterns and negativity about myself. The process helped me to see that really this was my father's problem, not mine. I felt very angry with him when my first insights about this came to light, then I was able to see so much sadness and disappointment in his own life. I feel like I have truly broken away from him now – his judgements and criticism. I don't have to be perfect and I give myself permission to enjoy myself more. More importantly, I now realize I really like myself and for the first time I am involved with someone in a non-abusive relationship.

In adults, making a lot of comparisons with other people is a sure sign of low self-esteem. People often measure the 'whole' of themselves by taking into account only one factor (such as their job) when there are a multitude of factors to take into consideration, which can be measured in different ways. They forget that many personal qualities and abilities cannot be reasonably measured at all. Ultimately, it is impossible to compare one person with another. It is rather like comparing an apple with an orange and asking 'which one is better?' Or asking whether an almond tree is 'better' than a cherry tree. Just like human beings, they have different qualities and too many factors to evaluate. People with high self-esteem tend not to compare themselves directly with others, because they are happy to be who they are and see many ways of valuing themselves and others.

I have seen many clients start to challenge and overcome the effects of negative feedback originating in childhood, by using their journal. Exercises in Chapters 5 to 9 explore self-esteem with regard to the entire family and offer techniques to help you find ways to combat early setbacks.

## The difference between self-esteem and confidence

We often use the terms self-esteem and confidence interchangeably. I consider them to be quite different. I believe that confidence is knowing that you have a skill in a particular field and you are able to engage successfully in that activity. It might be the confidence you feel in being able to drive, give presentations, play a sport or entertain people. It may be a confidence you feel with language or numbers, or a skill in playing a musical instrument or drawing. Confidence is a contributing factor towards self-esteem. Knowing and trusting you have ability in a particular skill helps you to value yourself. However, self-esteem is more complex and consists of more factors than merely confidence. Self-esteem is something deeper. It is the way you feel about your *whole* person, not only your skills and talents. It is something you wake up with in the morning and is a more general sense of well-being. High self-esteem is about feeling valuable and worthy just as you are *right now*, without having to prove anything. (A comprehensive list of the elements of self-esteem is given in Chapter 8, pages 74–5.)

I've always kept some kind of diary, on and off since I was about 15. I realise now that I used it in a very limited way – it was a muddle of random thoughts without any focus.

Since using specific journal exercises, it has opened up a whole new adventure of self-discovery. I feel like I understand myself much more than ever before, and most importantly, my confidence has definitely improved because I accept my thoughts, my feelings, myself more.

**Frank, retail manager, 43**

## The scope of a journal

There are many ways to keep a journal, depending on what you want out of it. You can use it to monitor your mood swings, to notice patterns in your behaviour, to monitor the way you are changing. You can record positive aspects and not only problems, dilemmas and difficulties. Your journal can be a resource file of achievements, strengths, new decisions and means of monitoring your progress towards goals.

In the next chapter we will explore more benefits of keeping a journal.

# 2

# Why writing is good for us

## The search for completion

Have you ever done a jigsaw, only to realize at the final moment that the last piece is missing? How frustrating does that feel? Can you recall the surge of satisfaction you might have felt when you were able to find that final piece and slot it into place?

We all have a need for completion and resolution. This applies to simple practical tasks, such as completing a jigsaw or crossword, as well as to situations involving complex emotions, such as understanding why we feel a certain way. Completion brings release, incompletion brings tension. We tend to dwell on unresolved personal issues in a bid to find resolution, just as we might search and hunt for that final jigsaw piece. We ask ourselves the same questions over and over, searching for some kind of answer which makes sense to us: '*Why* did my partner have an affair?' '*How* could my son be taking drugs?' If we fully understood and accepted these situations, these thoughts and questions would not keep pestering us. Once these questions are answered, or we adjust and reconcile ourselves to them, hitherto unresolved issues recede quickly. The issues are no longer incomplete and crying out for resolution.

Writing down our thoughts and feelings about disturbing issues, as opposed to merely *going over and over them* in our minds, is extremely beneficial in the search for resolution. When writing, our thinking is forced to slow down, because our hand moves slower than the speed at which our thoughts flash by. In writing we will be following an idea or train of thought to its conclusion through making sentences, whereas thoughts in themselves are often incomplete and fragmented. By writing out our thoughts through to their end point, we can begin to organize and manage them. In time, we can begin to understand them better and this in itself often leads to resolving the issues which are bothering us. Understanding and acceptance are the key processes involved in reaching emotional resolution and this is often achieved more quickly through writing, than going over thoughts in your mind.

When you place your thoughts and feelings on to paper, you are also physically separating from them. They are no longer inside your head, but in front of you on the page. This detachment often leads to a fresh way of seeing your situation. You may notice patterns of behaviours which take you to a deeper level of understanding and then you can begin to look at your options and choices within problematic situations. You may notice insights and possibilities where you thought there were none. When you *release* the problem from your mind on to the page, in the same way you might make a note of a telephone number, you no longer have to keep checking and rehearsing it in your mind. Once on the page, you can add to the outline of the problem, amend it and then try to get to grips with it.

Once you stop obsessing over a problem and clear it from your mind on to paper, you create a space where your energy can flow into a more productive examination of the problem. As a result, writing can be much more effective in reaching solutions than by purely dwelling on a problem.

## Three levels of exploration

Writing it all down gives us the opportunity to look at a situation from many angles and on different levels. In using a journal therapeutically, these levels include:

1 The *Emotional level* (self-expression: how something affects us and how we feel about it).
2 The *Cognitive level* (our thoughts about a situation, what sense we make of it).
3 The *Action level* (what we are going to do about it, the steps we could take).

Resolution can come about more quickly if we are aware of these different levels and can work on them appropriately.

### 1 The emotional level

The first level to address in the journal is the emotional one. The *emotional level* involves getting in touch with and finding words for the immediate raw feelings going on inside us. Some people find this very difficult because they do not *know* how they feel most of the time, and are certainly unable to *name* the feelings. Even after many years of self-development work, I am sometimes unsure about what I am feeling at any one time. I might know that something is not quite right, but I am not able to put my finger on how I am feeling and therefore I am unable to release or work through what is going on inside me. At those times I will turn to my journal to try to discover what my emotions are and how they are affecting me.

The emotional level starts with Exercise 2 (The 'agony aunt' method) in Chapter 4 (page 30). Exercise 1 (Getting to know your emotional inner self) in Chapter 3 (pages 26–8) explains how to practise finding meaningful labels for our feelings. When words fail us, or we prefer a more visual means of expression, drawing and image-making may be useful (see Chapter 10).

When using the journal at the emotional level we are making use of self-expression. The journal becomes a container for the way we are feeling in the 'here and now' or for recalling previous feelings. We are not analysing or attempting to understand anything, we are merely 'telling it how it is' and allowing our feelings, whether these are rage, sadness or excitement, to fully exist. In this way we are honouring our feelings and giving them room to be alive. We are moving our energy through these feelings rather than keeping them locked inside.

If you only use the journal to address this level, it is still likely to be beneficial to you. You may feel the 'clearing' benefits of self-expression and release and could gain some insights into your behaviour patterns. However, if you wish to take this further and work on developing your journal, you may find deeper benefits by using the cognitive and action levels. These levels go beyond self-expression and involve understanding and improving a situation.

## 2 The cognitive level

Once we have expressed and articulated some of our feelings about a situation, we can see things more clearly and objectively. Unless we access the emotional level first, we may find that our thinking is clouded by our feelings. This is the sensation of not being able to 'think straight'. Having worked through the first level of knowing *how* and *what* we feel, this second level focuses on trying to *make sense of things*. Exploration starts to take place through both reflection and self-awareness so that a new stage of acceptance, integration and understanding may be achieved. At this level too, a clearer overview, new perspectives and conclusions can be reached. Exercise 3: The four constructive tasks (Chapter 4, pages 35–6) shows you the steps involved in putting the *cognitive level* into practice.

## 3 The action level

After 'feeling the feelings' around an issue (emotional level) and reflecting on what we think about it (cognitive level) we may be ready for the next stage: *action*. This is the stage whereby we are ready to think ahead and to do some problem-solving. We are ready to look at choices, new possibilities, decisions and solutions. Now that we are no longer so wrapped up in the concern itself, we may start to outline steps we could take to deal more effectively with the situation. This is where practical movement in the form of action can take place.

Writing in itself promotes problem-solving, because in order to put down complete sentences and trains of thought, we need to spend more time thinking about the problem. We also have to simplify, state the bare bones of situations and go step by step in order for our writing to make sense. Writing forces us to keep our attention focused on one aspect of a problem at a time and encourages us to write in detail, to complete one idea, before we move on to the next. (Chapter 4, page 38, takes you through the 'problem-solving' process in more detail.)

## Using the different levels

When you use your journal regularly, you are likely to be shifting in and out of these three levels of exploration all the time. These three levels – *emotional*, *cognitive* and *action* – form the background to most of the exercises in this book. However, while it is useful to be aware of all three levels, you do not need to write within each level every time you use your journal for it to be effective.

Your need for working at any one level may change from issue to issue and day to day. Some situations may require a great deal of problem-solving, whereas other concerns may involve expressing your feelings as the essential element. You are likely to go back and forth between the different levels rather than go through them chronologically. In any one sentence, for example, you may touch on emotions (level 1) and try to make sense of something (level 2) and then go back to your emotions again (level 1). You might also notice that you find one level much harder to write within than the others, or that you are inclined to miss out a level altogether.

By being familiar and comfortable with writing on all three levels you are likely to get the most out of your journal. Chapter 11 shows a detailed example of progressing through all three levels using a 'worry map' (pages 104–8).

## The health benefits of keeping a journal

The release which comes when we get emotions out into the open is beneficial, not only for our mental health, but also for our *physical* health. Have you ever told someone a worry you had been keeping to yourself for some time? Did you feel a sense of relief and release when you did this? We usually feel as though a weight has been lifted from our shoulders when we unburden ourselves of worry, fear, guilt or shame. We can literally breathe more easily, relax our shoulders and feel at peace.

The journal can be part of this unburdening process even though no other person apart from yourself is involved. This is because you are allowing your feelings some kind of expression and not suppressing them inside yourself. To 'hold on' to worries or distressing thoughts requires physical effort, even when this is largely subconscious. We hold fear and anxiety as tension in our shoulders, throats, stomach and hands, for example. Sometimes unrelenting tension of this sort can lead to more serious medical problems, such as high blood pressure and stomach ulcers.

## Expression versus suppression

Many types of depression I see in my counselling practice are a result of someone having suppressed or 'pushed down' their feelings. They might feel ashamed of having certain feelings and thoughts (anger towards someone they love is a common example), or they may not feel anyone would want to listen to them, or could understand or accept them. They have not been able to let out their feelings and may even avoid facing these feelings within themselves. These 'depressed' people put on a brave face to the world, pretending everything is fine, but inside they are in turmoil. This kind of depression, where uncomfortable feelings have been blocked, tends to lead to a debilitating numbing down of all feelings. The person feels hollow and only half-alive. Apathy and feelings of pointlessness can then follow.

Janine's journal gives an example of how she suppressed her feelings:

**Janine, trainee nurse, 22**
When I had my termination two years ago, I kept it secret from everyone. I felt so ashamed and frightened of how people would react if they knew. My mother would have hit the roof. I had to keep it all bottled up. Through writing my journal, I realized that my periods of feeling low had begun to increase after that time, until I became deeply depressed two months ago. I didn't know what it was about at the time. I thought I was on a slippery slope to being really ill. Sometimes I couldn't get up in the morning and I would cry on and off all day.

After I started writing, I saw how I'd just pushed all my feelings down about the baby. I began to allow these feelings out in my journal and they were very powerful: hatred towards myself and God, grief, self-blame, sadness – everything – it wasn't easy. Afterwards I could see how brave I had been at the time and could value this in myself. I even dared to tell my best friend and she was brilliant.

I now feel that something is resolved. The sadness will always be there, but I've cleared out so much of the guilty shameful stuff. I'm feeling much better about myself and I am not depressed any more.

There is a hidden price of silence. When you express your feelings in your journal you will no longer be suppressing them, so you are likely to be less prone to this type of depression.

## The evidence for health benefits

In his intriguing book *Opening Up: The Healing Power of Expressing Emotions* (see Suggested reading), Dr J. W. Pennebaker, an American psychologist, explains how self-expression keeps us healthy. He demonstrates not only the therapeutic benefits of expressing oneself, but also makes links between self-expression, health and well-being. He argues that self-disclosure, whether through writing or talking, boosts our physical health as well as being good for our emotional well-being.

Dr Pennebaker carried out numerous experiments in the 1980s involving volunteers who were prepared to write openly about traumatic or upsetting issues in a controlled setting. One experiment with particular relevance here divided the volunteers into four groups. Each group wrote for 15 minutes a day for four consecutive days. One group was asked to write only about the *facts* of a trauma, the second group to write about the *facts and their emotional responses* to it in detail, the third group to write only about their *emotional responses* and the final group was asked to write only about *trivial matters*, such as the weather.

His findings showed that during the following six months after writing, the second group (who wrote about the whole event including facts and feelings) sought medical support 50 per cent less than in the months previous to writing. This marked decrease in reported illness did not occur in the other groups. Follow-up questionnaires were also carried out four months after the experiment to monitor the well-being of all participants. While those who had written in greatest detail about their traumatic experience had felt sadness and upset at the time of writing, they reported a more positive outlook, improved moods and greater physical health than those in the other groups (J. W. Pennebaker and S. K. Beall, 'Confronting a traumatic event: Toward an understanding of inhibition and disease', *Journal of Abnormal Psychology*, 95 (1986), pp. 274–81).

Further experiments led Dr Pennebaker to believe that we put ourselves at risk of a range of illnesses when we hold back strong feelings or thoughts and that it is beneficial to our short-term and long-term health to confront and express our deepest feelings. My professional experience often bears this out, with clients becoming less fraught and stressed when they begin using a journal to express themselves.

## Is a journal necessary?

I have outlined above some of the emotional and physical benefits of keeping a self-esteem journal, but you may be asking yourself whether you could get by without it. Is it something you *need* to do? Do you need to put in the effort that writing regularly would require?

If you are reading this book, the chances are you are interested in improving your self-esteem. More specifically, the self-esteem journal could be an invaluable help to you if you are experiencing any of the following symptoms:

- Feeling a loss of direction in life.
- Feeling unsure of who you really are.
- Carrying around pent-up feelings of irritability, anger or frustration.
- Feeling like crying at the slightest thing.
- Feeling 'numb', as though you are cut-off from your feelings.
- Feeling like everything is 'grey' and colourless around you.
- Feeling a sense of pointlessness, as though you are on a treadmill going nowhere.
- Feeling lonely, isolated, bored and cut-off from others.
- Wondering if you are 'depressed'.

When someone has low self-esteem, they are often out of touch with who they are and what they really want. They tend to pay too much attention to what other people think or want from them. They may feel stuck or trapped and often disempowered, because they are confused. What the world appears to demand of them and who they seem to be do not match up. They may end up blaming 'the world', but more often than not they end up blaming themselves and self-loathing can follow.

If you recognize any of the above symptoms and you feel you could be ready to deal with some of them, the tools in the self-esteem journal could be your starting point towards genuine recovery. The next chapter shows you how you can get started.

# 3

# Getting started

## The starting point

You can begin your self-esteem journal at any time in your life and the good news is that you do not need to make any changes to yourself first. You can start with exactly who you are right now at whatever stage you might be. Your self-esteem journal is designed to help you get to know and understand your 'inner' world so that you can deal with everything in the 'outer' world with more confidence. If you can begin to like yourself more, which is the ultimate aim of this book, this is likely to have a positive impact on your relationships, friendships, family, work and so on.

## Materials

Keeping a journal can cost you next to nothing. At its most basic all you need are some blank sheets of paper and a biro. You will need to find a size and format that suits you. Some people prefer to use an A4 ring binder, where they can insert extra pages, such as drawings, records of dreams or mind-maps (see Chapters 10 and 11). Others need something petite, which they can keep in their handbag or backpack, such as an art book, exercise book or Filofax. People who are familiar with computers may wish to type, rather than hand write their journal. You might prefer a ready-made page-a-day diary, or you may feel restricted by this. Consider when and where you are most likely to write in your journal, together with the style of your entries, as this could determine practical factors. The key is to find a format that suits you best and which allows you to write in a free and relaxed manner.

Here are examples of how some people got started:

**Lucy, fashion student, 21**
I write as soon as I wake up. I decided to get a chunky book filled with hand-made paper (from my local art shop) covered in Chinese-style

fabric. I use a cartridge pen with green ink, which makes my diary writing special and it differentiates it from all the other notes I make during the day using an ordinary pen. I like plain paper because I can include drawings and images from dreams, or create little charts when I am trying to make a decision about something.

*James, sixth-form teacher, 39*
I use an electronic organizer that has a mini keyboard for my self-esteem journal. It's really small, so I take it everywhere and write on the train and in my lunch break. I'm so used to typing everything that it feels natural and it suits me.

*The only time I can guarantee privacy for writing my diary is when I have a bath at the end of the day! As a single Mum with three young children, this is the only time I get to myself. I use a plain exercise book and waterproof ink! It works.*

**Julia, full-time mother, 28**

## Time and commitment

The progress of your journal will depend on the amount of time you can spend writing each week and how committed you can be to the process. Like any process, you will need to put in some effort before you experience the unfolding benefits. At first it is preferable to write every day if you can, in order to become familiar with tuning in to yourself and exploring how you feel. In this age of busy lifestyles, however, this may not always be possible. Ideally writing for 20–30 minutes each day, or every other day, gives you continuity and helps you to work through the issues in this book steadily and step by step. There may be times when you want to spend longer periods reflecting on a particular issue, and then times when you need a total rest from writing. Finding a regular time to write, such as first thing in the morning, or last thing at night, will keep up the momentum and sustain the flow. After a while, you may start to acknowledge the issues you are ready to face and the amount of time you are prepared to give to them. If you only have two minutes to spare every day, you can still keep a 'pillow book' (for details of this and other quick journal tools, see Chapter 12).

We all need to stop the 'busy-ness', reflect on our lives and review our futures from time to time, otherwise we can feel we are on a treadmill, lacking meaning and direction. By keeping a journal you provide a space each day or so to stop, truly listen to yourself and check where you are heading. Your journal time will be dedicated entirely to you; a time to honour your thoughts and feelings. It is a private time in which to connect to your inner world without all the demands and distractions of everyday life. During your journal-time you can withdraw from the rest of the world and concentrate on you and put *you* firmly back in the centre of your life.

Most people I know who have been introduced to the self-esteem journal incorporate it into their lives as a long-term self-development tool. While at times you may want to take a break from your diary-keeping and consolidate your insights without it, emotional issues will always be on the horizon. You can never be 'done and dusted' with this kind of work, because you are constantly growing, changing and unfolding and there will always be new issues to face, or previously unresolved ones that re-emerge. Your journal is your opportunity to work through problems, to learn, grow and move forward.

## Under lock and key

Your self-esteem journal will be different from any other book ever written and may be with you for life, so you will want to find ways of looking after it and respecting it.

Privacy and secrecy are extremely important in keeping a journal. You will be revealing deep and intimate feelings in your self-esteem journal, which you may not want anyone else to know about, least of all your nearest and dearest. You might not feel able to be truly honest in your writing, if in the back of your mind you fear discovery and exposure. You will need to find, therefore, a place that will be as safe and private as you can make it.

I used to buy journal books that had a little lock and key. Now I have so many jottings, drawings and sheets of image-work, that I keep them safe in a lockable box. I also write a preface to every file or book, which reads: 'In the event of my death or incapacity, please respect my privacy and destroy these private papers without reading them.' I have also appointed someone I trust who will look for these papers and destroy them when I am no longer around. You will need to find your own ways of ensuring the privacy of these most confidential records.

## Being honest

In order to write honestly about your feelings and thoughts, you may need to dig deeply into your emotions and challenge yourself. It is all too easy to operate on a superficial level in our lives and it would be easy to do this also with our journals. We often keep up a façade that 'everything is fine' when clearly it is not. We might even hope that the problems will go away by themselves if we ignore them. Avoiding or denying painful issues that face us might help us to keep going in the short term, but in the long term such issues need to be resolved. Through using this book, you can learn to give yourself space to face difficult issues and teach yourself the tools you need to work through them.

In order to use the journal most effectively, you will need to consider being prepared to do the following:

• Be willing to express yourself.

- Allow feelings to surface (some of which may have been long buried).
- Be as honest as you can be.
- Be prepared to dig deep and feel some pain or confusion.
- Be willing to challenge yourself.
- Devote some time most days to your inner self.

The benefits of approaching your writing in this way can help motivate you to go beyond the superficial. You will soon discover your own approach to working therapeutically, depending on the amount of time you have and your level of commitment.

## Finding a language for your feelings

Before you can express how you feel in your journal, you need to *know* how you feel. If you are not used to being aware of how you feel, it will probably be difficult to turn to the first blank sheet of your journal and write about your emotions. People are often unaware of how they are feeling at any given time. If someone were to ask, 'How are you feeling right now?' – would you know?

For a variety of reasons, many of us have become detached from our feelings and go through life never exploring, sharing or fully understanding our inner emotional world. This can leave us slightly detached from other people. It also leaves us detached from ourselves, because we may never know what we need or want, never know and accept all aspects of who we are. When we are out of touch with our feelings, it is as though a part of us is hidden or cut off from *ourselves*, so we do not feel complete or whole. This can lead to a lack of self-esteem because only parts of our whole self are known, valued, accepted or loved. Other parts of us are left 'unchartered', often viewed by ourselves with suspicion and doubt, through lack of understanding.

Being 'out of touch' with feelings is common in the following cases:

- Adults who, as children, 'grew up quickly' in order to support a parent who suffered trauma, illness, divorce or the death of a spouse. The child would have put her or his own needs aside because of the overwhelming neediness of a parent.

- Those who spend a great deal of energy trying to gain approval from other people, so that the focus is less on how they themselves are feeling, but more often on how others might be feeling.
- People who have been badly hurt emotionally and who attempt to 'switch off' their feelings because they see them as painful and dangerous.
- Those who have been brought up in families where feelings are kept hidden and are seen as messy and disruptive. In such families, feelings are rarely explored or discussed. The 'stiff-upper-lip approach' stems from this kind of environment.
- People who focus on being intellectual and can 'talk about' experiences but who do not allow themselves to feel, or be in touch with their emotions. In this way, feelings are unfamiliar and to be distrusted, whereas 'thoughts' are measurable and clear and more highly valued.
- Those who keep themselves busy all the time, so that they do not have to stop and face their own feelings for fear of finding out they are unhappy.
- People who choose to work with other people's feelings in a vicarious way (such as counsellors, social workers, psychiatrists), because they are uncomfortable with their own emotions.

### Finding ways to express feelings

In order to become familiar with our feelings, we need to be comfortable identifying and acknowledging them and we need to develop a language that adequately expresses them. No matter how uncomfortable and distressing our emotions are, they are an integral part of being human. Our feelings are going to be forever with us, so we need to find ways of working with them rather than against them.

### Exercise 1: Getting to know your emotional inner self

This exercise is aimed at helping you to experience, identify and label feelings, so that you can develop the skill of expressing emotions in your journal.

1   The list below contains a selection of commonly experienced emotions and states of mind. Most of them are difficult and uncomfortable feelings that we often try to avoid. Select five of them at random and imagine how each feeling usually affects you and when and where you felt it last. See if you can recognize in a personal way each of the five feelings you have selected.

*Feelings, emotions and states of mind*

| | | | |
|---|---|---|---|
| despondent | distressed | useless | fulfilled |
| numb | needy | disengaged | threatened |
| anxious | spiteful | satisfied | outraged |
| relieved | insignificant | miserable | bitter |
| elated | disturbed | lost | hurt |
| nervous | embarrassed | aggressive | joyful |
| misunderstood | bored | powerless | trapped |
| unworthy | lonely | angry | rejected |
| ashamed | agitated | unloved | envious |
| vulnerable | out of control | abandoned | irritated |
| guilty | sad | resentful | fraudulent |
| confused | frustrated | frightened | insecure |
| directionless | jealous | | |

2   Imagine how each of the five feelings you have selected affects your body, paying particular attention to the effects you experience in your abdomen, solar plexus, stomach, chest and throat. We usually experience feelings in a physical as well as psychological way. You may, for example, experience being 'frightened' as tightness in your abdomen. Notice which parts of your body are affected by each emotion. Refer to the list of 'body-felt sensations' below, to notice some of the physical responses that can accompany emotions. Which physical sensations do you associate with the five feelings you chose? (Add them if they are not on this list.)

*Body-felt sensations that often accompany emotions*

| | | | |
|---|---|---|---|
| tearful | floppy | migraine | apathetic |
| tired | cold | buzzing | nauseous |
| can't breathe | itchy | floaty | ache/pain |
| clenched fists | sweaty palms | headache | tight |
| sore | tight throat | dizzy | feverish |
| frail | sweating | backache | hungry |
| heart racing | wobbly | unclean | explosive |
| shaky | neck-ache | | |

3   Referring to both lists now, circle the feelings and sensations you experienced most during the last week. Go more deeply into the words you have chosen and write a sentence or two about how they affected you. What did these feelings really mean for you? (For example, if you wrote 'hurt' you might realize this also meant that you 'felt to blame', or 'felt vulnerable'.)

4   How did you deal with these feelings? How did you take care of yourself when you had them? Did you allow yourself to express them, or did you pretend the feelings were not happening and attempt to push them away? Write a little to explore these questions.

One way we can develop self-esteem is to take very good care of ourselves when we are experiencing difficult emotions. The way we *talk* to ourselves (in our continuous internal self-talk) can seriously influence how well we take care of ourselves when we are emotional. (This is explored further in Chapter 5.)

By getting to know your feelings better, you can learn to be open to a full range of emotions, to respect them, value them and start to understand what they mean to you. Then you can recognize that they are there for a reason: you can learn from them, use them to enrich and develop yourself and grow through them. Your self-esteem journal can be the place where this inner journey begins, as you listen to yourself and write down whatever you come across in your inner world. Your next task, outlined in Chapter 4, is to find your own voice.

# 4

# Finding your own voice

Your self-esteem journal is your private place for cutting through the 'dressing up' and getting down to the bare bones of who you *really are* and what you *really feel*. It is a place where you can start to give a voice to hidden and suppressed feelings and reveal the genuine you. In time, through finding a language and through the habit of using words to express your innermost emotions, you may then feel able to share some of these feelings *with others* and develop intimacy, authentic contact and support. By talking and listening honestly to yourself first, you are preparing to talk and listen to others with more understanding and compassion.

In this chapter we will be working through each of the three levels of journal writing identified in Chapter 2: *emotional*, *cognitive* and *action*.

## The 'agony aunt' method

Once you have had some practice at identifying your feelings using the exercise in the previous chapter, you are ready to take this a stage further. For this exercise, you need to write for about 20 minutes with the intention of 'emptying out' every troublesome thought and feeling that is currently bothering you. I call this the 'agony aunt' method, where you use your journal to help you to clear away lingering worries, niggles, troubles, doubts, problems, anxieties and unresolved issues. It makes full use of the *emotional level* of self-expression and can be the starting point of your writing now and at any other time. The 'agony aunt' method can be the first stage in feeling more at peace with yourself and building self-esteem. You can make the transition from feeling confused or overwhelmed with a jumble of concerns (low self-esteem), to gaining clarity, taking control and moving forward (high self-esteem).

### Exercise 2: The 'agony aunt' method

The essence of this exercise is to keep writing regardless of whether or not you feel you are making sense. You do the 'agony aunt' exercise by focusing on all your troubled feelings and thoughts and allowing them to spill out on to the page for 20 minutes at the start or end of every day. Rather like opening a floodgate, this is an opportunity for you to allow all your emotional burdens to be released. If you get stuck, try to keep writing about what you are experiencing at that very moment ('I feel stuck – I don't know what to write about – I don't know what I'm feeling – this is silly'). As you keep writing you are likely to go beneath the surface of your thinking into something deeper. You may discover feelings you did not even know you were carrying around with you.

For this exercise you do not need to be concerned with grammar or spelling, or whether what you write has continuity. You can jump around from one topic to another or keep repeating something which needs to be expressed. Try to avoid making it sound interesting, clever or sophisticated or writing as though you have an audience. If you do this, you will be censoring what you write. The point is to 'empty' all the clutter out of your head by putting it on the page in its raw state, so that you start or end the day with a fresher state of mind.

## The vacuum cleaner image

Our mind is rather like a vacuum cleaner. It 'sucks up' worries, half-formed ideas, unresolved problems, untackled concerns and stores them all. Then we go over and over these worries in our mind without getting anywhere with them, or resolving them. Or we might have troubled sleep and disturbing dreams where fears and anxieties keep bubbling up from deep within. There might be recent events which have made us feel angry or resentful, which we have not told anyone about or worked through. There may be new or ongoing problems which we can hardly bear to face. This is all the 'stuff' that goes round and round in our heads which never seems to get sorted out.

Our concerns and problems are all the bits of 'dust' we accumulate, and this can leave us stressed, burdened and stuck. We need to keep emptying that 'vacuum cleaner', to clear the contents regularly out of our mind, so that we feel lighter and have more clarity about our lives. Many people I work with use the 'agony aunt' method as an ongoing daily exercise to help them find out what is hidden beneath the surface of their thinking. By using this method you will also be getting to know yourself better, which is one of the factors in developing self-esteem.

While this method is an excellent means of clearing out day-to-day worries and muddle, it can also help you to get an overview of what is going on. Quite often, you may be so involved in responding to a particular event, or feeling burdened with certain intense emotions, that you lose sight of the broader context. Things can then get out of perspective or balance. By writing about what is bothering you, until you get to the point where it all feels out in the open, you can step back, take a breath and consolidate. You are likely to see things which you could not notice before, because you had your head down, buried in the thick of it.

Here is an example of the 'agony aunt' method:

**Stephanie, aromatherapist, 31**
I'm feeling really awful today – not sure why – just flat and fed-up. It seemed to start when I got up this morning, but I don't know, I just feel really useless and stupid for feeling that way. I had a good day yesterday with Paul, so I don't think it's anything to do with him. It's as though I, I can't find the words for it, fed-up is partly what it is, but it's not all of it. I feel like hitting my fist down on the table. I can't be bothered to write this – it all seems so pointless. How am I supposed to know what's wrong with me? I just feel like this. I've been feeling like this so often recently, ever since ... yes, I think that's it – ever since I said I'd move in with Paul. There's something not right about it and I don't know why ...

In this extract, Stephanie struggles to find and name what she is feeling. Then something emerges for Stephanie from her writing that she did not know before. Once she started to trace back her feelings, she could see *when* things had changed for the worse. At this stage, she still does not know exactly what the trouble is, but she knows what it is connected with. She has clues now, a starting point, to further her enquiry and find out more about what is troubling her.

Most people I know who have tried this exercise tell me that something significant usually emerges even from a seemingly sketchy and vague starting point. This is explained below by Sophie who had been keeping this kind of journal for only three weeks:

**Sophie, music student, 21**

I was very surprised when I first started keeping a journal. I had no idea all these thoughts and feelings were buzzing around in my head, until I started focusing on writing it all down. I feel a lot clearer now. I think a number of things had been getting on top of me and weighing me down without me knowing what was happening. Now I feel more clarity about what these worries are and I know what I have to work on.

If you are not sure how to begin writing using the 'agony aunt' method, here are some ideas:

- Start by writing down 'At the moment, I feel …' and keep writing.
- Use 'I feel' statements rather than focus on other people or events.
- If you are unable to identify any particular feelings, start with a blank page and free-associate on anything whatsoever which comes into your mind and see where it leads you.
- Ask yourself, 'What is *really* going on for me, right now?'
- Reflect on what is 'working' and what is 'not working' in your life.
- Ask yourself, 'What's the worst part of all this?'
- Identify areas you want to improve and change.
- Write from an angry, frightened or usually 'unheard' or denied part of yourself.
- Try to notice anything you might be avoiding and name it, even if you do not explore it any further at this stage.
- Try to notice things about yourself, your patterns and habits.
- Record any dreams and fantasies.
- Reflect on your own personal needs and what you truly want from life.
- Reflect on how you deal with problems, setbacks and anxiety.
- You could include the positive as well as the negative.
- If you wish, you could list your accomplishments each day, even small achievements.

## Your first week of journal writing

While we will all use a journal in different ways, you might like to consider doing the following after writing for a week:

1 Reflect on whether you feel less burdened and more clear-headed. Have you slowed down? Are you less stressed?
2 Read over what you have written. Are your issues any clearer or do you have a clearer overview of your situation? Looking back can help you to realize that things have stopped bothering you or that you might have let go of something. This can give you confidence during difficult times that feelings can pass and situations which once felt overwhelming can gradually fade or transform themselves over time.

You may prefer to discard what you have written without reading it. This is still likely to have benefits, as you will be letting go of concerns and confusion and providing a release for your troubles. You might want to ask yourself why at this stage it is important to discard, rather than keep, your writing.

In the beginning your writing may seem disjointed, unruly, self-pitying and messy. This does not matter. The 'agony aunt' method of journal writing is purely a means of getting something off your chest. It is about allowing your feelings out on to the paper, without trying to make your words sound impressive.

## The first benefits

Increased self-esteem and self-acceptance are the overall benefits of expressing your deepest feelings – you are making friends with yourself, because you are starting to listen to and understand yourself. If you were to keep a journal using only this 'agony aunt' method for a number of weeks, the other likely benefits can be:

- Gaining immediate release and relief, because you are getting everyday matters off your chest (like a weight being lifted from your shoulders).
- Clearing away the clutter of niggling, often half-formed thoughts.
- Bringing into the light, hidden and suppressed feelings and thoughts.

- Becoming acquainted with your turbulent emotions and needs.
- Becoming less frightened by your feelings, because you have labelled them and are getting to know them.
- Getting clarity about what is going on, gaining perspective and seeing how you might have got some things out of proportion.
- Getting worries out of your head and on to paper where you might be able to see some choices and possible courses of action.
- The possibility of making better decisions because you can see a bigger picture.

With practice at expressing your feelings in a safe place, you are likely to be able to find appropriate words for explaining confusing thoughts and feelings. By exposing yourself only to *yourself*, you will see what it is you are dealing with. Many of the people I see for counselling say they realize they have to admit something to themselves first, before they can then face issues head-on. They need to cut through their own denial and avoidances in order to acknowledge that there *are* problems in the first place.

Malcolm found that writing in a personal way was harder than he thought it would be:

**Malcolm, sales adviser, 52**
I thought keeping a journal would be a doddle – I am good with words and I like writing. However, the first thing I realized was how much I was dressing everything up, trying to make it sound impressive and interesting. I realized I was doing this in life all the time – trying to sound better than I was, to get noticed. I hadn't realized that I hadn't been genuine with others or myself for ages – if ever. Having to cut through the presenting, approval-seeking part of me was very difficult, but I started to be able to voice honest feelings for the first time in my self-esteem journal. I could see a much more solid self emerging, which was both scary and very exciting.

## Four constructive tasks

In Chapter 2, the second level of journal writing was referred to, called the *cognitive level*. This is where a constructive approach comes into play, taking our emotional outpourings (the *emotional level* used in the 'agony aunt' exercise) one stage further.

A constructive approach is beneficial for adding meaning and understanding to your journal entries beyond a purely cathartic and clearing process. It gives you the opportunity to bring your *thinking* and *analysis* into the process. The *cognitive level* can help you to:

- Put issues into perspective.
- See a broader picture.
- Check whether you are overreacting.
- Be more objective.
- Look at concerns more rationally.
- Make sense of things.

When things make sense, we usually feel more confident in dealing with them, which fosters our self-esteem. By understanding a situation you can shift from confusion and feeling out of control, into clarity and feeling empowered. Furthermore, understanding a situation can lead to acknowledgement and acceptance of feelings, which also build self-esteem. When you see the whole picture with more understanding, you can start to see that you have certain feelings for good reasons. In this way you will be valuing your feelings, rather than dismissing them.

### Exercise 3: The four constructive tasks

When you are familiar with the 'agony aunt' method and can do this easily and quickly each time you use your journal, then add the following four constructive tasks to your writing:

*1 Sum it up*
At the end of each entry add a conclusion or summing up. This is a way of drawing together what you have written and getting an overview. For example, you may realize that your writing focuses on one particular person, or you may notice that you are not adjusting well to certain changes. Try to encapsulate your situation using only a few words or go to the start of your entry and give it a 'title' in the same way that a fiction writer might give a title to a chapter of a book. You might wish to ask yourself, 'What is all this about?' You are attempting to step back and get a broader perspective on what is going on for you.

*2 Search for themes*
To get a sense of what the main issues are, or those which keep recurring, look for themes and patterns in your writing. You can do this when you have made several entries over a period of time. For example, you might want to underline sections of your writing where you refer to different aspects of the same problem, or where you see situations which remind you of similar situations from the past.

*3 Who is doing the writing?*
Ask yourself which 'part' of you is doing the writing. Is it a childlike part (perhaps confused or vulnerable)? Is it a grieving part (mourning for something which is lost)? Try to name which aspect of yourself is driving the writing.

*4 Prioritize*
Decide which aspects of your concerns are urgent and must be dealt with immediately and which ones can stay 'on the back-burner' for a while. Go back through your latest journal entries and make a separate list of the issues you are currently facing, then number them in order of importance or urgency. Which ones must you deal with immediately? Which ones can wait?

This helps you to prioritize the issues you are facing, so that you do not feel overwhelmed with them all at once. You may have thought originally that everything had to be resolved straight away, when in fact some issues can be left for a while, and may even benefit from being approached after further reflection.

The example below shows Rosie's first attempt at addressing the four constructive tasks in one of her journal entries. The section following the example highlights each of the four tasks as they have been addressed by Rosie in her extract.

**Rosie, full-time mum, 41**
My anger has taken over everything and it has definitely helped to get it out on to the page. My son has made me feel rage like I've never felt it before. When I look over what I've written, I realize that I feel a great sadness too. While I am feeling so much hatred for my son right now, I also see how gutted I am. I can't believe it has come to him walking out like that – so there's this shock factor too. I realize from my writing that the worst part of it is that he didn't try to talk to me about it. It leaves me feeling so sad – that he couldn't tell me how he felt. I thought our

relationship was better than that ... I'd call this period of my life 'when we stopped communicating'. I never saw this before. This is definitely what I need to look at first – the whole communication breakdown between us.

## How Rosie used the four constructive tasks

*My anger has taken over everything ...* (Task 3: Rosie identifies which part of her is driving the writing.)

*When I look over what I've written, I realize that I feel a great sadness too.* (Task 2: Through rereading, Rosie sees other themes in her writing – she had not realized before that she felt 'sad', as well as 'angry'.)

*While I am feeling so much hatred for my son right now, I also see how gutted I am. I realize from my writing that the worst part of it is that he didn't try to talk to me about it.* (Task 1: Rosie is getting a new perspective on her feelings and she now knows the worst part of this issue.)

*I'd call this period of my life 'when we stopped communicating'. I never saw this before.* (Task 1: Rosie gets an overview and finds a description to summarize what is going on.)

*This is definitely what I need to look at first – the whole communication breakdown between us.* (Task 4: She pinpoints the issue she needs to address first.)

Rosie was able to acknowledge and accept a range of feelings she had been experiencing towards her son and to see that their relationship had been suffering from a lack of communication. She was moving on from blaming her son to seeing that she might also have played some part in the problem. Rosie did not have any answers at this stage, but she was starting to explore the bigger picture and saw that communication between them was the area that needed to be addressed first. By unravelling her situation through her writing, Rosie began to understand more about what was going on and her self-esteem increased, because she soon discovered that there was a way forward with her difficulty.

You can apply the four constructive tasks in any order you like. They are designed to help you to get an overview of your preoccupations, to gain some clarity about how you are feeling and what you might need to do next.

## The 'problem-solving' process

Following the four constructive tasks, you can progress to the third level, the *action level.*

This is the problem-solving stage, which allows you to move on from expressing your feelings and understanding your situation more, to finding strategies for moving forward. It is good for our self-esteem to work on something in a productive way, as it allows us to see we have some power and control. This stage gives you the opportunity to mull over potential courses of action which could lead to improvements or solutions to your difficulties.

### Exercise 4: The 'problem-solving' process

Here is the problem-solving process for you to try, step by step:

*1 Identify control*
Starting with your most urgent issues, identify the areas where you think you have some control.

Jane was going through a hard time, feeling overwhelmed by her personal circumstances. Among other issues, she was fearful about going into hospital for a knee operation, she was in the stressful process of selling her flat and she felt smothered by nagging and intrusive phone calls from her mother. Jane assessed her level of control as follows:

> *Medical operation* (no control), *selling the flat* (some control), *my mother phoning me all the time* (no control).

When you make your own assessment of control, try to look at different aspects of the situation to *search for* control where it seems you have none. You might need to challenge yourself here. Upon reflection you might see that you do have some control after all. Jane (above) found that in her issue 'my mother phoning me all the time', she had more control than she thought. She saw that she could be more assertive towards her mother when she rang, without being unkind. She could make clearer boundaries about when and how long she would be available to chat and she could avoid her mother's prying questions by taking the lead and discussing subjects she felt comfortable with.

*2 Brainstorm*
Identify *all* possible courses of action you could take to make even the smallest improvements with your problem. Brainstorming is very powerful here. The process of brainstorming is to think of every conceivable idea which might improve things, no matter how insignificant, unsuitable or unlikely these ideas may seem.

We often seek solutions in a limited way by dismissing many of them as impossible when *something* about the idea could have been taken further. In brainstorming, quantity, not quality, is the first aim. To begin, the flow of ideas needs to come from a place of creativity, not practicality. You can review your ideas and judge how realistic and workable they would be at a later stage. If you judge too soon, you may miss an idea which might have worked (if it was, say, coupled with another idea). For example, I often hear people say during the brainstorming process, 'Oh, but I would never do it that way – I'd have to be a different kind of person to do it that way.' So I ask them to include the courses of action they might take, if they *were that different kind of person*. So, try not to box yourself in during this brainstorming stage. Generate as many 'wild and wonderful' options as you can. You could even share this process with someone you trust who knows of your situation, in order to formulate more ideas.

*3 Identify action*
The next stage is to search through your brainstorming ideas to see if any plausible courses of action emerge. Use your journal to weigh up the relative pros and cons of your options. Choose the most suitable ideas and write them out. You might want to come back to them after a break to see how you feel about them with a fresh state of mind.

*4 Define smaller steps*
Sometimes we get stuck at the point when we have discovered possible courses of action, because the changes we could make seem too big and difficult. The ideas for improvement might seem useful, but we do not know where to start to put them into effect. It is important therefore to break down your most likely solutions into smaller steps. You are aiming to end up with small manageable progressions towards your goal. Consider what action you can take this week towards resolving your issue. Then look at what you could do *today*, even if it is only to find a relevant telephone number or to find something in a reference book in the library or on the internet. Bring your possibilities into the present moment as far as possible. Where will you start? What could you do in the next *hour* towards improving your situation?

Adding a problem-solving aspect to your writing helps you to gain control and a sense of moving forward, which greatly enhances self-esteem. You can use your journal in this way to search for strategies for improvements at work, in your relationships, domestic issues and so on. By keeping an ongoing record of the issues you are working on you can review and monitor your progress.

## Turning worrying into problem-solving

It is easy to assume that when we spend a lot of time on something, we are making headway with it. This is not always the case and is certainly not true if we are merely worrying about something. Worry tends to go round and round without resolution, building anxiety and panic. It wastes a lot of time and energy and it ultimately does not get us anywhere. Relentless worrying can contribute to low self-esteem, because it can leave us feeling impotent and powerless. When we worry, but do not take any action regarding the cause of the worry, we can feel like a victim of outside circumstances and can stay stuck in this passive position.

Through your journal you have the opportunity to express the worrying (*emotional level*), but then to transform it into something more productive which can be dealt with (*cognitive* and *action levels*). With increased self-awareness, you can begin to notice when you are worrying, express it, then challenge your worrying in order to turn it into 'problem-solving'.

Problem-solving is a *productive* process which helps you to define the action required in order to alleviate the problem. In this way it is an antidote to worry and it is also a boost to self-esteem. By engaging in problem-solving you are empowering yourself by giving yourself options and choices about how to make changes. You are no longer a passive victim, but taking matters into your own hands. This builds self-esteem, because it gives you more control and shows you that you can make a difference. When you next find yourself worrying about something, try the following exercise.

**Exercise 5: Turning worrying into problem-solving**

1 Ask yourself what *exactly* you are worrying about. Use the 'agony aunt' method to express every aspect of the worrying situation you are facing. You may be concerned about a health scare, a fear of someone dying or a fear of a partner having an affair or leaving you. Or it may be a less acute worry about work, a friendship or your future. Write out your deepest fears from every angle, including all the 'what ifs' and worst possible outcomes. Try not to minimize your concerns, but instead express the entire 'awfulness' of the situation. Write about this worry until you have exhausted it. You may need to revisit this stage of the exercise over several days in order to express every perspective of this worry.

People often say to us 'don't worry', but this can lead us to bottle up our feelings. When someone says 'don't worry' it can really mean 'don't burden me with this' or 'you're being silly'. Our worries will be there anyway, bubbling away under the surface, and by writing them down you allow them to be released without burdening someone or being judged by them. By taking the time to air your worries fully, you are honouring your feelings and respecting yourself.

2 The next step is to summarize the worry in one sentence, for example: 'I am worrying about my constant headaches,' or 'I am worrying about being made redundant.' If you have several worries which are linked to each other, separate them out and do this exercise with each one.

3 Does the worry belong to today/next week/tomorrow/yesterday/ last year? Pinpoint the moment in time associated with this worry. Dealing with a worry which has its source in the past may require a different approach from a worry about something which has not yet taken place. We often dwell on something from the past which is over and done with. Rather like a videotape, we keep replaying a difficult incident in our minds, conjuring up all the same feelings of vulnerability, embarrassment, fear and so on. In its extreme, this replaying of traumatic incidents could be diagnosed as post-traumatic stress disorder. (If you have recurring nightmares, panic attacks, flashbacks and constant edginess, then it would be advisable to consult your GP.) Once you have an exact time-frame for your worry, move on to the next step.

4 If the worry is about something in the *past*, then ask yourself what would have to happen for you to lay this issue to rest. Do you need to confront someone or something? Do you need to forgive someone or forgive yourself? Do you need to brainstorm ways to resolve some unfinished business?

An extract from Sarah's journal addresses these questions about a past event causing worry:

> **Sarah, student, 20**
> I can't get those hurtful words my sister said to me out of my mind. It happened six months ago, but it still seems like yesterday and I just go over and over that day, trying to work out what I did wrong. I now worry that I am a bad person because of her reaction to me. I've now decided to write a letter to her, I might not even send it, but I want to write down everything I've gone through since then. I might even arrange to see her again. I know it will be really difficult, but I've got questions that have never been answered and never will be unless I face this.

Notice that Sarah turned her worrying into problem-solving during this extract at the point at which she decides to write a letter to her sister. She realizes what she needs to do to address this worry connected to the past. What would you need to do to face your worry?

5 If the worry is about something in the *future*, ask yourself if there are any practical steps you could take *now* to help your situation. Can you find a way to prepare yourself, such as rehearsing what you might need to say to somebody or checking something out, or asking for help, or for someone's opinion? Or can you let go of the problem for now and promise yourself you will come back to it at a time when you *can* do something about it?

Glen gives us an example of finding practical steps to deal with a future event causing him worry:

> **Glen, gardener, 24**
> I am worrying today about a dentist's appointment next week. I hate the dentist and I'm scared stiff. However, there is nothing much I can do about this right now, so I will try to let it go for the moment. On the day itself, I will do some deep breathing and ask a friend to go with me. In this way I will be doing the best I can for myself.

6  Worrying is usually a fear that you will not be able to cope with a situation in the future, or a feeling of pain or unfinished business about something which has occurred in the past. Ask yourself what is the worst that could happen surrounding your worry and then state how you would cope if this took place. Complete these sentences:

a)  My most feared outcome is ...
b)  I will cope with my most feared outcome because ...

Sarah (page 42) completed these statements as follows:

a)  My most feared outcome is ... 'that there is something wrong with me and that I am a bad person'.
b)  I will cope with my most feared outcome because ... 'I intend to get to the bottom of the row with my sister. I want to know what I am supposed to have done that was so terrible. Finding out cannot be worse than this awful not knowing.'

7  For worries about something in the future, you can try this exercise. Close your eyes and visualize the scene where you are dealing with the difficult situation. Imagine that you and any others involved are relaxed and coping. You are breathing deeply, knowing that you are surviving the problem issue (the problem issue may still involve sadness, anger or physical pain, but imagine that you are tolerating it and remaining calm). Above all, you survive.

8  If you are an ardent, 'full-time' worrier, allow yourself only 20 minutes every day to do your worrying. During this period do nothing but seriously worry. Sit down with your head in your hands and 'fret'. If you begin worrying at other times, make a note of your worry and then save it for your next 20-minute allocation. If you have had your worry period for that day, save your worry for tomorrow's session. If you want to think about the problem outside your specified worry time, refer to the 'problem-solving process' on pages 38–40 and make sure that you *brainstorm solutions*, so that you are doing something productive.

When you turn worrying into problem-solving several things can change:

- You become empowered, because you are actively doing something to improve your situation.
- By taking action you may be able to change the outcome of your worry from your worst fear into something more positive.
- You start to build your confidence in dealing with problems, trusting you can cope and think them through. This gives you confidence for facing and dealing with future problems.
- Your self-esteem is likely to increase, because you are taking responsibility and moving your position from being passive to proactive.

Remember, once you have fully expressed your feelings, the antidote to worrying is to start building strategies for tackling the problem as it appears in the present. Worrying does not solve anything, but problem-solving does. The energy you waste in worrying can be turned towards making choices, decisions or taking action – all of which build self-esteem. In the next chapter, we will look at the role of self-awareness in developing self-esteem.

# 5

# Techniques for self-esteem

## Self-awareness

An essential step in building self-esteem, as it is in making any sort of change, is to work out what needs to be improved. This chapter helps you to seek out where your difficulties with self-esteem lie, so that you know where to focus your energy for change. The key to this is 'self-awareness'.

If you do not know what needs to change, it is hard to find ways to move forward. One important function of your journal is to help you to develop self-awareness, so that you get to know yourself better and become aware of how you behave and express yourself. Then you can identify some of the things you would like to do differently.

Self-awareness is crucial in making improvements to your self-esteem. It is about 'noticing' aspects of yourself, but doing this in a way that is not self-critical. Self-awareness is not about finding fault or looking for means to blame yourself. It is a process of bringing your thoughts, emotions, underlying beliefs and habitual behaviours into your consciousness so you can examine them more clearly. This 'noticing' is a process of standing back from yourself, *in a non-judgemental* way, and watching yourself, gently and lovingly, as though you were observing another person you care about. It is a means of noticing all the elements that make up who you are with open curiosity and from a place of compassion.

In day-to-day life, we can spend a lot of time losing ourselves in external distractions. Life can feel like a treadmill or rat race, and what we really need to do is to stop, get off, tune in to who we are and refocus on where we are heading. With so many outside influences and activities going on in our lives, we might be left with little awareness of what we want, how we feel and what we need to help us live fulfilled lives. Perhaps we also spend a lot of time doing what we think other people want and as a result we lose touch with who we are: our own opinions, values, abilities and plans for ourselves.

Not only does self-awareness help us to uncover areas we might want to change, but it also helps us to take time to get to know ourselves. How can we appreciate and value ourselves if we do not know who we really are? Self-awareness helps us to begin to discover our true natures and get a deeper sense of who we are.

## The benefits of self-awareness

The benefits of self-awareness can be summarized as follows:

- Self-awareness teaches you to stand back from your thoughts and be detached and separate. It reminds you that you 'have' thoughts, but that *you are more than* your thoughts.
- The method of listening to your thoughts in Exercise 6 on page 48 is the basis of various forms of meditation. It is beneficial in helping you to cope with anxiety and overactive thoughts, often associated with stress or panic attacks.
- Self-awareness helps you to know yourself more and see which unhelpful patterns of behaviour you find yourself repeating.
- You can also notice aspects of your personality which you enjoy and cherish. By putting you, your feelings and thoughts in the spotlight you can recognize your strengths and positive qualities as well as highlighting areas you might want to improve.

The main functions of self-awareness with regard to self-esteem are twofold:

1 To explore what you *do*. By noticing your responses and patterns of behaviours you can discover more detail about situations you find difficult, uncomfortable or which lead to self-sabotaging cycles. At first, you will probably do this only after the event has happened. With practice you may develop awareness in the actual moment itself, so that you create the opportunity to modify your actions and responses, there and then (see the 'self-esteem cycle' in Chapter 8, page 76).

2 To explore how you 'talk to yourself'. The importance of the inner self-talk to self-esteem was mentioned in Chapter 1. This

is the function of self-awareness we will focus on in this chapter, where we will evaluate the content of our inner self-talk in more detail.

## Tuning in to your inner self-talk

Our behaviours and the way we respond to outside events often stem from what we are telling ourselves in the monologue we hear inside our heads. A negative statement to ourselves, such as 'I am so stupid', is likely to lead to different behaviours when compared to a more positive statement, such as 'I am doing really well'. The first statement could lead us to feel ashamed and unworthy, to withdraw from other people or perhaps avoid them altogether. The second statement could result in approaching others with confidence and openness, leading to a warm sense of belonging.

When you pay attention to your inner self-talk you can notice whether it helps or hinders you. Self-awareness will help you to notice the nature of your inner self-talk and to find out whether it tends to be more positive or negative towards you. Once you are familiar with the nature of your inner self-talk and how this might be affecting your self-esteem, you can start to make changes to it.

Jerry describes his early attempts at noticing his inner self-talk through self-awareness:

*Jerry, fitness instructor, 20*
I began to listen to the inner chit-chat I have with myself – especially with regard to relationships. When I was getting ready for my first date with Sandra, I was telling myself that I didn't look right and that she'd find me unattractive. I was panicking about what I would say on the way to the nightclub and I could hear this loud voice inside my head saying: 'She's way out of your league, man – she's not going to be interested in you.' It was like a voice mocking me. It was very hard just to listen objectively without getting even angrier with myself for putting myself down. I noticed that this sort of thing happened a lot and it made me see how distorted my inner dialogue was, how biased it was against me – I wasn't giving myself a chance!

## Preparing to change your negative self-talk

By improving the way you talk to yourself on a daily basis, you can greatly increase your self-esteem. The three steps below will prepare you to challenge and modify how you speak to yourself:

- Step 1: Develop *self-awareness* – monitor and become aware of your inner self-talk.
- Step 2: Develop *deeper self-awareness* of the *manner* in which you talk to yourself. Find out whether it is a mostly positive or negative voice.
- Step 3: *Exploration* – find out where the negative voice comes from.

Steps 4 and 5, which complete this process, can be found in the next chapter.

Let's look at the first three steps in more detail:

### Step 1: Self-awareness

#### Exercise 6: Listening to your thoughts

In terms of your 'inner' world, there is a lot more going on than perhaps you might think. When you try to 'listen to yourself' what do you hear? Can you tune in to the multiple thoughts, ideas, flashes of memory and to-do lists which are flitting through your consciousness all the time? Try this exercise to help you to tune in to your daily 'self-talk':

1 Find a time in a quiet place where you can be alone and undisturbed for about 5–10 minutes.
2 Begin by getting comfortable and closing your eyes.
3 Take four or five deep breaths. Notice the air rushing in, filling your lungs. Let each out-breath be slightly longer than the in-breath, fully emptying your lungs. Leave a little gap before the next in-breath.
4 Now draw your attention to all the sounds going on around you. There may be a clock ticking, or traffic, voices, music – just notice these sounds and let them come and go. Do not put any effort or energy into thinking about them. This is your awareness being focused outwards. You may not have realized just how many sounds were going on around you.

5 Then begin to listen to your thoughts and focus your awareness inwards. Just notice each thought and label it as it comes and goes. We usually get caught up in a thought and go along with it until the next one. In this exercise, however, the intention is to notice the thought, register what the thought is about and let it go. An image for this process might be to imagine that your thoughts are small sticks and leaves carried along by a river and you are standing on the riverbank watching your thoughts float by.

For example:

Our usual thinking: *OK, I'll stay quiet and listen to myself for a minute ... I feel fidgety ... I must remember to get some stamps ... I'm not sure what I'm supposed to be doing in this exercise ... I feel achy and can't be bothered ... I must remember to post Dad's birthday card ...*

This exercise: *Oh, I must get some stamps* (notice the thought and label it) ... *Ah, there's a thought about stamps* ( let it go and refocus again on watching your thoughts).

6 Carry on doing this. Each time a thought comes up, notice it, label it and let it go. A jumble of thoughts may come up together. Try not to follow them through, but avoid berating yourself if you get lost in your thoughts for a while. Keep bringing yourself back to being the detached observer and centre yourself into listening again.

This is a difficult process to do at first, because we are so used to getting caught up with where our thoughts and feelings lead us. One moment we might be thinking about what to buy for dinner and the next we find ourselves remembering a past hurt or something we did wrong a week ago. We do, however, have the ability to stand back and watch what is going on.

It is important to remember that we all have these inner 'voices'. Listening to this self-talk is not to be confused with any kind of schizophrenia or mental disorder. In self-awareness, we are simply listening to our own continuous background commentary on our life and how it impacts on our self-esteem. There is nothing dangerous in raising our awareness. The self-talk is going on within us all the time anyway and we are merely bringing it into our consciousness.

The next stage is to try and listen to the *manner* in which you talk to yourself during the day. This is what helps to determine high or low self-esteem.

## Step 2: Deeper self-awareness

### Exercise 7: Focusing on your inner self-talk

1 Try to 'listen in' to how you respond inwardly to situations. What sorts of things are you saying to yourself *about* yourself? Do you encourage yourself and praise yourself? Do you speak to yourself respectfully? Do you put yourself down? Do you expect too much, or too little from yourself? Your daily chatter will carry on subconsciously most of the day, so rather like tuning in a radio, you need to actively listen to how you are responding to your actions and behaviours.

2 Try to listen to yourself during a whole range of activities: at work, at home, when you are travelling, when you go to the shops, when you engage in conversations with others, when you are alone, when you make decisions to do certain things. Tune in particularly when you have done something well or when you have made a mistake or not done as well as you had hoped. Listen to how your inner self-talk responds to these circumstances.

Notice the tone, manner and words used by this inner voice as these can have an enormous impact on your self-esteem. Listen for words in your inner self-talk like 'should', 'ought' or other words of judgement or criticism. If you have low self-esteem you will probably hear many critical responses to your behaviours. You might hear statements like: 'There you go, being a failure again,' 'You've made a complete fool of yourself,' or 'No one's going to be interested in you.' These responses can leave you feeling ashamed, humiliated and 'not good enough'. Most of the time you are probably unaware that these destructive messages are being fed into your consciousness throughout the day. If these messages are cruel, this is going to be damaging to your self-esteem on a daily basis.

If you have high self-esteem, you might hear statements such as, 'You coped well with that situation,' 'You can be proud of yourself,' or 'It's OK to make mistakes.' These kinds of responses are likely to leave you feeling confident and good about yourself. For the time being just notice what comes up for you. We will be doing more work on transforming your inner self-talk in the next chapter.

## Positive and negative self-talk

Having learnt how to tune in to your inner self-talk, you will now be in a better position to evaluate how helpful and encouraging this inner monologue is to you. When you tune in to your self-talk, do you hear mostly positive or negative statements about yourself? Which voice tends to dominate? Which one is loudest? Remember you are evaluating the 'voices' inside, not yourself. You as a person are separate from the monologue going on within you.

Low self-esteem is often associated with more negative self-talk than positive. This negative voice can, however, be challenged and changed. First, we look at where this negative voice might have come from.

## Where do the inner 'voices' come from?

Your inner self-talk is like a tape recording inside your head con-sisting of large numbers of 'messages' you have been told about yourself. These 'inner tapes' contain statements about ourselves and our worth that we have heard from influential people such as parents, family and teachers, during our upbringing. During those early years of childhood and adolescence we are subconsciously getting a sense of who we are and we do this by taking in how others respond to us. The world is rather like a mirror, letting us know how we are perceived. Using the responses and feedback we have received from people over the years and regarding this as our 'evidence', we subconsciously create our self-identity. If someone important to us picked fault, we might see ourselves as 'bad' or 'dif-ficult'. If they ignored or neglected us, we might regard ourselves as 'unlovable'. Likewise if we were praised and celebrated, we could see ourselves as 'worthy'.

We will have internalized the attitudes significant people had towards us and whatever we heard will become the basis of our inner 'tapes'. This becomes the foundation of our inner self-talk. What we probably failed to realize was that feedback from others might not have been valid. We accepted it as 'truth' about ourselves, when it may have been a distorted projection made by another person, rather than a fair and unbiased response to our behaviours. In this way, we can see that our inner self-talk consists of other people's subjective beliefs about us. As such, it is not likely to be an accurate mirror of who we really are. Our inner self-talk, for the most part, is therefore *not our own voice* and it is probably far from being a reliable means of establishing our self-worth.

## Step 3: Exploration

### Exercise 8: How to identify the source of your inner self-talk

Once you have started to get to know the nature of your inner self-talk, try using your journal to answer the following questions:

1 Over a period of a week or so, which negative statements keep popping up?
2 Who do you associate with the most common ones?
3 Do you hear several voices representing different kinds of comments on your life? Or do you hear one consistent voice?
4 Try to identify the predominant critical or negative voice. Is it a male or female voice?

When I do this exercise in counselling sessions, people often say, 'But it's just *my* voice.' Remember that because we have been hearing this voice (or voices) for many years, we will have transformed it into our own voice. We assume that this commentary on ourselves has been developed by us alone. Can you trace the most frequent statements back to when you first heard them? How old were you then? Do you associate them with school, friends, home or somewhere else?

5 Is the voice old or young? Does it remind you of anyone? Can you put a face to the voice you hear most often?

The journal extract below describes Derek's first attempt at identifying the source of his negative inner voice:

### Derek, IT project manager, 27
When I began to tune in to the self-talk inside me I got confused. I was hearing only my voice telling me that I wasn't good enough. Only when I tried to focus more carefully and used my memory to track down the history of these statements did it hit me! These words belonged to a

female voice – to my mother; they were the words she used to say to me when I was a kid – always preferring my older brother to me, always putting me down.

Suddenly I could see her face when I heard this critical voice inside me and I knew it was her.

Laura recalls her discoveries about her negative self-talk:

**Laura, trainee life-coach, 33**

When I grasped the idea that I might have picked up lots of conditioning about myself from early influences, I listened in to what my inner self-talk was telling me. I realized that I had several nasty, hurtful voices, but I couldn't relate them to my parents or family at all. Then I realized that they came from when I'd been bullied at school. I had completely forgotten about it, although it went on when I was 11 to 14 years old. My inner critical voice seemed directly related to the things those horrible girls had taunted me with – being too small, not being clever, not having friends. It formed the basis of all the things I was telling myself as an adult.

In Chapter 6, we will explore how to challenge the critical voice within and develop nurturing and supportive inner self-talk.

# 6

# The turning point

In Chapter 5, we identified the first three steps in exploring your inner self-talk. To complete this process of transforming the negative voice into a positive one, take a look at the final two steps below:

- Step 4: *Challenging* the negative voice to search for the hidden motives behind this voice.
- Step 5: *Replacing* the negative voice with a positive, loving voice.

## Challenging the critical voice within

If you are suffering from low self-esteem the chances are that you hear stronger critical or negative 'voices' within you than supportive, positive ones. These 'tapes' from the past create the basis of your current self-image and you will probably expect to be treated in accordance with these negative statements. Likewise, you might tend to dismiss anything that does not fit your view of yourself (hence the reason why people with low self-esteem find it difficult to receive compliments). Because you have internalized negative statements about yourself, you are likely to find ways to reinforce them unless they are challenged. Steps 4 and 5 show how you can defeat the negative voices inside you.

### Step 4: Challenging

#### Exercise 9: How to challenge the critical voice within

Here are some ways you can challenge the negative 'tapes' you have been playing to yourself all these years:

1  When you notice the negative voices, start to say to yourself, 'Ah, there's that voice having a go at me again.' Use self-awareness to

step back from the voice and see what it is trying to do to you. Would you talk to a best friend in this way? If not, why are you accepting this amount of criticism when you talk to yourself?

2 Find a face to fit the most common negative voice and imagine having a conversation with this person. See them in your mind standing before you and ask why this person feels the need to treat you like this. Remember that as an adult, you have lots of experience, skills and wisdom that you did not have when you were a child or teenager. At the time when you first heard these statements, perhaps you were much younger and not able to challenge the person who was criticizing you. Now you have the opportunity to question what those critical statements were all about.

3 In your mind, ask what was going on for that person in their life that they needed to put you down. You may realize that the critical person was jealous or envious of you. Perhaps they were so busy trying to cope themselves, they did not have enough time for you. Consider what the motives might have been for the person who originated these damaging comments. Perhaps they were taking something out on you because of issues in their own life. Maybe they were lacking in self-esteem themselves. Maybe they said something they did not mean, in the heat of the moment. Perhaps they were even trying to protect you from something, but doing this in an unhelpful way. By questioning the motives and state of mind of the person who delivered the negativity, you can start to question the validity of their statements about you.

4 If this person is still living and available to you, you might consider asking them these questions in person if it feels safe enough. They may give you a new perspective you never knew about. They may throw light on circumstances in the past that allows you to see their responses in a different way. They may not even realize that you took something to heart that they never meant in a hurtful way.

5 Challenge the statements. Find evidence for yourself that proves the negative statements are untrue for who you are in your life now. For example, if someone criticized you in the past for being lazy, you might find lots of ways to show that in the present time, you are far from lazy. This statement is therefore out of date.

6 Consider whether what was said had more to do with the person who delivered the criticism, than you. Did this person project on

to you something that they could not tolerate in themselves? For example, someone may have convinced you that you were unattractive, but they were actually feeling unattractive themselves and (perhaps subconsciously) wanted to pass their pain on to you.

7   Whatever the origins of the negative messages, once you have challenged them and believe that they are out of date, invalid or unjustified, imagine *giving them back* to the person who said them. Imagine each message as an unwanted parcel and visualize giving it back saying, 'This is not true and I do not want it any more.'

8   If you cannot find a face to fit the negative voice, imagine a cartoon image to suit the kind of voice you hear. You might imagine an angry little gnome or a tiny green devil. When we associate the voice with a cartoon picture, it can lose its power. It begins to look foolish and exaggerated. When you next hear this voice, associate it with your cartoon character. Then you can poke fun at it for a change and diminish its control over you.

9   Try 'turning down the volume' when you start to hear the critical voice. Imagine retuning the radio station in your mind to find a more supportive voice for yourself.

10  Identify one hurtful statement that has stayed with you over the years. Sometimes someone can make a throwaway comment only once, and it stays with us all our lives. I remember, in my early teens, finding out that a teacher had made a cutting remark about me behind my back. He had said, 'She's hardly Miss Personality!', which deeply hurt me at the time. I carried that statement with me for many years afterwards. Every time I let myself hear that comment in my mind, my self-esteem took a knock. Much later, I was able to use the techniques above to challenge it. Only then could I see that this teacher was insecure himself and lacking in his own social skills. I realized that the statement he made said more about him than about me. I found evidence in my own life to show me that people did find me interesting and amusing. The statement was no longer valid in my life, so I was able to wipe it from my inner tape.

Write out a hurtful statement word for word alongside the name of the person who you believe originated it. Do this for all the statements you are unhappy about and challenge them using the steps above.

## Developing a nurturing voice

If you have discovered that your inner critical voice is 'louder' and more obvious than a supportive one, there are ways to develop a more nurturing voice for yourself to counterbalance it.

### Step 5: Replacing

#### Exercise 10: How to develop a nurturing voice

Here are some techniques to replace the negative voice with a positive one:

*1 Remember someone who cared*
Try to remember anyone from your past who had kind supportive words to say to you. It might be a grandparent, an aunt or uncle, a teacher, nurse or an older sibling.

Close your eyes and imagine that this person is there with you now. Even if this person has passed away, conjure up the memory of them. Use a photograph if this helps you. How might this person encourage you at this stage in your life? What things would they say to reassure you? Try to hear the quality and tone of their voice and to see the kindness in their face as you hear the sorts of statements they said in the past.

Referring to any of the negative comments that continue to bother you, how would this supportive person challenge this particular negative view of you? What words would they use? Imagine hearing their caring words and write them down. Carry these words around with you if you wish and refer to them at times during the day when you are slipping into negative thinking about yourself.

*2 Be a loving parent to yourself*
If you have difficulty remembering anyone who supported you as a child, imagine that you are a loving parent hearing someone make critical accusations to a child you care about. How would you protect and defend this child? Can you transfer some of this care to the child part of you? If you did not receive enough loving support from your parents, this allows you as an adult to give to yourself what you missed out on as a child.

*3 Find the opposite*
Choose one of the most damaging negative statements you hear in your self-talk and write down the opposite. For example, if you hear, 'You're so stupid sometimes,' turn this around into 'You're really clever sometimes.' How does that feel? Who could you imagine actually saying this to you? Give yourself a moment to 'hear' them saying it.

Remember that we tend to focus on responses we get from people that reinforce our self-image. If our self-image is negative then we will tend to hear only further negative statements, or interpret responses as negative. Positive statements will go over our heads and we will not pay attention to them. Once we get a more balanced self-image by developing the nurturing voice within, we are likely to find ways of reinforcing it and be more able to accept positive statements made about us in the present.

Clara described her experiences of developing a kinder inner voice in the extract below:

### Clara, publishing assistant, 25
When I tuned into my inner self-talk I realized I was hearing all the things my stepfather had said to me as a child: telling me I wasn't clever or pretty enough, telling me he was ashamed of me. I'd taken all this in and was living with it every day, even though my stepfather died years ago. I decided to try to create another voice inside which would take better care of me, and I called her 'Mrs Tea and Sympathy'. She reminded me of my Nan. Every time I heard my inner negative voice, I tried to call on Mrs Tea and Sympathy to see what she had to say in response. I saw a big round woman in a striped apron and I imagined her putting her arms around me. She allowed me to feel vulnerable without feeling weak. She allowed me to have fears without feeling that I was useless and to be angry without feeling guilty. It completely transformed the way I felt about myself to have this alternative approach inside me. It was one of the major breakthroughs that led to improving my self-esteem.

Clara felt she had missed out on the nurturing statements she would have internalized growing up, which would later have become part of her adult inner supportive voice. Instead she faced her stepfather's internalized critical voice every day. By developing the image of 'Mrs Tea and Sympathy', she could listen to her needs better, instead of obsessing about improving herself. This helped her to develop self-acceptance ('I am OK just as I am') – an essential element of self-esteem.

People with low self-esteem tend to have an under-developed inner nurturing voice. Can you find space inside yourself for a nurturing and supportive voice? At which times in particular would you call on this voice to bring you solace and encouragement? For example, you could invite this voice to help you when an interview does not work out, when you feel rejected by someone or when something deeply disappoints you.

*4 Your inner support team*
Many native American Indians believe in having imaginary contact with people they admire as their inner resource of support and strength. When they do not have a real-life support network of friends and family around them, they *imagine* the security they would like to feel. They conjure up the voices and attitudes of people they know, or have heard about, who have great courage and integrity. They visualize people they greatly respect and admire who would support them and stand up for them. Then they inwardly call on them for help and support when they are feeling lost or afraid.

You can try creating images of the sorts of people you would like to have in your team of internal supporters. These can be real, fictional or historical figures who would believe in you, give you good advice, accept you just the way you are and have qualities and strengths you could draw on. You can imagine these people when you hear your negative self-talk. You might want a number of allies to support you when facing different challenges; someone supportive when you are feeling low, someone who has great drive when you want to get a new project off the ground or someone wise when you need to make a decision.

Make a list of four or five personal allies who could be supportive to you in your life today. What qualities do these characters represent? You can choose supporters and allies from people in history (they can be dead or alive), from real people in your childhood who valued you and listened to you, from television, films, books you have read, fictional characters and so on. Choose any character at all where you think, 'It would be great to have someone like that around – they'd be really supportive.'

Close your eyes – imagine one of them sitting or standing with you now. Silently introduce yourself and make contact. Try to picture their eyes, their face, and the appreciative way they look at you. What do you think they might say to you? Do they have any guidance or advice right now? If they were to describe the things they like about you, what would they say? Then say goodbye for now and know that you can call on them at any time. Open your eyes and make notes in your journal. In particular, write down their advice to you, so that you have something concrete to help you.

Even though you may have a circle of good (real-life) friends, having a resource of 'inner helpers' is valuable at times when friends are not available. My supporters change from time to time depending on what I need. I have had characters from television programmes and films because they were heroic, spirited or determined. I have called upon a former college tutor in my mind to ask him for his opinions. Athletes, Tibetan gurus, psychologists, writers of self-help books have all been part of my imaginary team.

If it seems ridiculous to 'create voices' inside your head, remember that there is already a 'voice in your head' created from critical statements you have heard from people in the past. Why not turn this negative voice into positive encouragement?

*5 Affirmations*
One way of developing positive self-talk is by using affirmations. These are positive statements made about yourself in the present tense, usually starting with 'I am ...' Some examples are: 'I am a loving and caring person,' 'I deserve a loving relationship,' and 'I am good at what I do.' By making these positive statements regularly you counterbalance the negative statements you habitually say to yourself.

In her book, *Feel the Fear and Do It Anyway* (see Suggested reading), Susan Jeffers explains that it is not essential to believe the affirmations at first. Experiments have shown that experiencing any kind of 'positivity' creates an uplifting energy in the body. Furthermore, by speaking to yourself with positive statements you may find that you gradually 'take them in', in the same way as you 'took in' all the negative statements – it is the same process.

Think of some affirmations now and make a short list of four or five. You could make a section in your journal devoted to an ongoing list of helpful affirmations. Affirmations need to be framed in clear, positive statements in the present tense for the best impact. Here are some more ideas:

I am strong and in charge of my life.
I am capable and confident in what I do.
I am an interesting and lovable person.

I am complete within myself and have everything I need inside me.
I have many positive qualities and gifts.

If after tuning into your self-talk, you hear mostly negativity, it is not sufficient to try to ignore the negative voice. All this does is push the negativity to one side for a while, so that it can attack you in another moment. You need to challenge and discredit the inner negativity so that it starts to lose its power over you. When you develop a more nurturing self-talk your self-esteem will improve, because you will be treating yourself with more respect, acceptance and love.

In the next chapter you can find techniques to expand your journal methods to get to know and understand yourself better.

# 7

# Going deeper

Many of us find that, although we may be burdened with worries, there are times when feelings seem too private to share with even our closest loved ones. We cannot bear to talk through personal details with others for fear of embarrassment or shame, or perhaps we fear we will not put across our feelings adequately. Concerns might seem too difficult, painful or dangerous to be scrutinized even within ourselves and are therefore kept locked away. Because these hidden feelings are never opened up or looked on with love, they never shift perspective or get challenged. They lurk in the shadows of our deepest selves, sometimes for years, creating layers of fear, guilt or weakness which drag down our self-esteem. It is for times like this when your journal can be most therapeutic.

When you begin to write out your feelings you can often reach into these shadows and bring to light feelings you had previously not admitted to yourself or had driven deep within yourself. You may even think you *know* what you are feeling, but when you put words on paper and describe your emotions in more detail, you can touch on material you did not know was there and peel away the layers, bringing clarity and understanding.

Great relief can be achieved by simply asking yourself, 'What's wrong?' at times when you feel muddled or anxious. You need to do this in a loving and gentle way which respects your feelings and gives them space.

Sadly, it is often with a less encouraging frame of mind that we approach ourselves. Instead of a kind, supportive voice asking, 'How are you really feeling right now?' a critical voice can emerge saying, 'What on earth's the matter with you? For goodness sake pull yourself together,' or 'What right have you to be miserable when so many people are worse off than you?' This critical voice drives you away from listening to yourself and away from exploring what is bothering you. Then you are left not only with the original feeling, but also a feeling of guilt for *having* the feeling in the first place. That is why it is important, not merely to ask yourself open questions about your hidden feelings, but to ask them in a loving way, without judgement.

## Writing from the child part within

One way of accessing hidden feelings is to try to set the adult part of you aside and write from a much younger self. This will help you to get a fuller picture of your feelings, because you will be removing the adult influence which can get in the way. This adult part is likely to be doing the following:

- *Justifying* – 'My low mood is just because I'm tired.'
- *Avoiding* – Distracting yourself by being 'busy', focusing on other people's problems or using something to alter your mood, such as alcohol, so that you do not have to focus on the real issue.
- *Moralizing* – 'I shouldn't be thinking of myself at a time when my mother is so ill.'
- *Minimizing* – 'It will pass, it's nothing, it's silly to feel like this ...'
- *Rationalizing* – 'I've got so much going for me, I shouldn't be depressed' (trying to talk yourself out of your feelings).

When accessing an inner 'child' voice you can go beneath the adult distractions and reach the true essence of what you are feeling. The examples below illustrate the difference between writing from the 'adult' and writing from the 'child' voice inside us.

Jenny wrote from her adult voice:

**Jenny, financial adviser, 39**
I am feeling very upset because my mother has been taken ill. The thing is, I am finding it very hard to cope with her on my own, but I feel terrible saying that and I should be just willing to give over my time to her. I must put on a brave face and get on with it.

As she wrote, Jenny's feelings of anger were pushed away, because she felt guilty about having them. These feelings stayed locked up inside her and eventually led to bitterness and resentment. Guilt tends to stop our genuine feelings in their tracks. We put a lid on feelings of resentment or frustration because we think having them makes us a bad person. The problem is that the genuine feelings are going to be there anyway, only they will be unacknowledged and suppressed. This means you are hiding part of yourself, not liking part of yourself and therefore causing your self-esteem to suffer.

Martin wrote from his child voice:

> **Martin, commissioning manager, 33**
> My dad coming to stay has totally put me out. I don't want him here. I am angry that he has invaded my space – I need my freedom. Privacy is so important to me. How dare he turn up unannounced and assume he can settle in with me. I feel totally suffocated …

Martin gave himself permission to write for several pages about his feelings towards his father, many of which he had never acknowledged before. He allowed himself to *feel* these difficult feelings of rage and accepted them in himself (they were still inside him, shaping his thoughts and feelings, whether he acknowledged them or not). While the adult part of him might have persuaded him not to be 'so selfish', by staying with his childlike feelings about his father and airing and clearing them, he was able to move to a better emotional place. This experience was about honouring his feelings more, enabling him to take care of himself. At a later stage he was able to find ways to address his feelings with his father.

### Exercise 11: Writing from the child part within

This is a useful exercise when you are feeling emotional or upset. In order to write from your deepest truth about your feelings, try accessing the childlike part of you and ask the adult self to step aside. This can give you permission to vent difficult emotions such as anger, rage, grief, loss and fear without justifying or rationalizing. This is not easy to do straight away, so the following ideas might help you:

1 Find a photograph of yourself when you were much younger, between the ages of five to ten years old. Look closely at this picture, notice what you are wearing, notice what is in the background. Try to conjure up the feeling of being in that picture – what would you be able to touch, smell and see if you were to shrink down in size and step into the photograph? Try to associate the difficult feelings you are experiencing with this younger self you once were.

2 Using your non-dominant hand, write from this child part of you. This will replicate some of the awkwardness of learning to form letters and words that you experienced as a child and it can 'take you back' to an earlier time.

3 Focus on writing your strong feelings until you have exhausted them. Children often get very fired up with a feeling, such as anger, and they storm about, throw tantrums, howl, scream and so on. They do not apologize for a feeling or play it down, they give it everything they have got. When the feeling has been fully expressed and is out of their system, they are usually able to move on and feel a completely different emotion, such as joy, very quickly. Write out your feelings until you have got all of it out on to the page. If you need to be physically expressive when you write, you can do this too, such as thumping cushions, stamping your feet, banging your fists and so on.

4 If you find yourself slipping back into your adult self, try to notice this and set the adult part on one side again. You can always come back to writing from the adult part of you later on. You will know the adult is trying to take over when you find yourself using words like 'should', 'must', 'ought', 'duty' or when you feel a sense of being 'selfish'. Children are self-centred; up to six or seven years old they are only capable of seeing the world through their own experience. They are still learning to empathize, project or imagine what other people might be thinking or feeling. The reason for inviting you to write from this part of you is to put you and your feelings back in the centre of your life. It does not mean that you will become a selfish person. It is encouraging you to redress the balance lost in low self-esteem where you do not acknowledge, honour or respect your own feelings sufficiently.

In the above examples, Jenny carried resentment around for a long time, which caused her guilt and pain and prevented her from showing genuine love towards her mother. Martin, on the other hand, having privately expressed and acknowledged his feelings about his father, felt sufficient self-acceptance and courage to face his father in person and work through some long-held hurt with him.

## Re-parenting the child within

In the previous chapter we looked at developing a nurturing voice to take better care of us and how this is often easier if we imagine ourselves being a loving parent to our own child-self. Here we look at this child part in more detail.

Many people I see for counselling seem to have a long-held raging battle inside themselves between their 'child' and 'adult' selves. This struggle comes about because of feelings which seem to originate from a younger, smaller, more vulnerable self. They often see these childlike feelings as holding them back from being adults and causing them to feel 'weak', 'stupid', 'incapable' and so on. But just because we are adults does not mean that we never experience some of the feelings we had when we were younger. We do not leave every aspect of that child behind – he or she is still living within us.

One way to envisage this is to imagine a set of wooden dolls which open up revealing smaller and smaller dolls inside. Using this metaphor, each layer can represent the different life-stages we have been through: baby, infant, child, teenager, young adult and so on. We might only see the outside adult shell, but these other younger selves are there none the less. We do not suddenly only have 'adult' feelings just because we have become adults – we are still carrying around all the other selves and other elements that make up who we are. If we try to ignore or deny the feelings which seem to stem from these younger parts of us, we will not feel completely whole or integrated and will have a sense of struggle and disharmony.

One client, Mark, told me he hated the part of him which he called his 'little boy'. This part of him often seemed to hold him back from fully grasping opportunities in his work as a sculptor. He saw this little boy part as 'weak and pathetic' and got angry with himself, instead of taking care of this part in a loving way. By the end of our sessions together, Mark had started to pay attention to the feelings of this 'little boy' and to see that those feelings stemmed from insecurities he had experienced with his stepmother as a child. He listened to those feelings and started to understand where they came from. He also began to accept them as part of himself. He started to respond to his little boy with comfort instead of disdain. This meant he was less angry with himself and he gave himself permission to deal with situations differently. When he was feeling vulnerable, he would take time to find out why this was happening and to give himself inner encouragement and support. This was how Mark described the change in his approach:

*Mark, sculptor, 26*
Now that I take care of my childlike feelings, my adult and child self share a more harmonious existence. I have even begun to realize that the child part has something to offer the adult in me. My little boy is creative and spontaneous in a way that my rational, practical adult self is not. Now my little boy can bring inspiration to my art work and the adult part takes care of the frightened little boy during those times when I feel lost or confused.

## Learning to identify a younger self within

Mark learnt to separate the different voices inside himself and to recognize the emotional 'child-derived' responses. He did this by paying attention and monitoring his feelings. If you find yourself overreacting to situations or expressing what seems like inappropriate feelings, these may stem from a younger you. Common 'childlike' feelings are blind rage, tantrums, jealousy, confusion, vulnerability, hurt or fear. These can be debilitating to you as an adult, if you do not have a way of responding positively to them. Such feelings are likely to emerge when you are tired or stressed, as your usual resources for coping with them will be diminished.

### Exercise 12: Identifying and re-parenting your child self

Use your journal to work through the following:

1 When do you overreact to situations? When did you last respond to a situation with feelings which were inappropriate for the situation? Are your feelings sometimes overwhelming? Write about recent examples.

2 Which of those feelings seem very 'deep'? (this is often a clue that these feelings have been with you for a long time). Which ones seem to be 'all or nothing' or 'black and white', such as 'I am all bad,' 'This will never get better,' 'I will be like this for ever'?

3  Try to label all the feelings you associate with deep overwhelming situations.

4  What patterns are there in the kind of situations which trigger these strong feelings (for example, scenarios when someone criticizes you or when you feel left out)? List the situations which commonly bring about these extreme reactions.

5  Choose one situation and the feelings associated with it. Do you get a sense of the age you were when you first had this feeling or the source of it? (It can be useful to find early photographs of yourself to help jog memories of being a child. This can help to identify difficult events and how you were treated.)

6  Now visualize yourself at the age associated with these recurring deep feelings. Can you imagine what you were wearing at that age and what your appearance was like? Try to see this younger self in your mind or use a photograph to remind you.

7  Can you understand why the child you were then became so upset? Can you see any similarities with the circumstances that upset you now?

8  Now imagine the words a comforting parent would give to a child in the same situation. How might a caring parent respond to a child suffering in this way? Write down the actual statements you would like to hear, as well as any actions which might go with them (such as, 'It's OK to feel angry – you are confused and nobody has explained what's going on to you properly.' The parent then hugs the child and allows the child to feel upset).

9  Can you imagine offering this kind of support to yourself when you next feel a childlike feeling? Can you listen to that child part of you to see what it needs from you? Can you respond to these needs by offering yourself time, space, permission to have the feelings, encouragement, loving words or whatever it takes to feel better? In some cases all you might need is for the child part of you to be heard and acknowledged.

If you are with other people, you might need to find somewhere where you can be alone in order to calm yourself and offer the child part of you comforting words. If you cannot easily remove yourself there and then, you might need to promise yourself that you will take some time later to address it.

Use this process of re-parenting yourself with other situations from the list you made in question 4 of this exercise.

Jilly explains how re-parenting helped her:

*Jilly, personal assistant, 33*
I could not understand why I became so insecure around my boss and why he made me feel so small. When I explored my feelings at work, I realized that they reminded me of being around my dad when I was younger. Dad always made me feel so stupid and insignificant and I realized there was something about my boss which pressed exactly the same buttons even now. Instead of telling myself to 'grow up', I started to feel very sad for the 'little girl' in me who felt belittled. It made such a difference to understand why I felt so feeble around my boss and to treat myself with kindness, instead of beating myself up. I am now able to see how different my boss is from my dad and I'm amazed that we are getting on better.

Once you are able to recognize these kinds of overreactions and identify the feelings as belonging to a younger self, you can see how it feels to respond in a loving way to this part of you. You will then be doing for your child self what a considerate parent would be doing. In this way you will be accepting yourself more, integrating your many inner selves, being loving towards yourself and therefore building your self-esteem.

In Chapter 8, we will reflect on how we measure self-esteem and explore some of the factors which influence our level of self-esteem.

# 8

# Getting to grips with self-esteem

How do we measure self-esteem? Which areas of our lives need more self-esteem?

Some people find that their self-esteem is good in some areas of their lives and less good in others. Susie, for example, felt very confident and capable in her work as a project manager, but awkward and self-conscious in social settings, especially in large groups. Derek, however, felt totally comfortable with groups of friends, but felt nervous and inadequate at work. Tamsin felt self-assured about her personality, but insecure about her looks.

## The self-esteem ratings chart

In which areas of your life do you most lack self-esteem? Is your level of self-esteem the same in each part of your life? Are there areas where you feel you have less self-esteem than in other areas? Try the exercise below to help you define the different levels of self-esteem you experience. It will help you to see in which life-areas you need to do most work and also in which areas your self-esteem may be better than you thought.

### Exercise 13: Rating your self-esteem

Indicate how you rate your current level of self-esteem in the following life-areas by copying out the chart below and circling the number which most applies. Use the scale of 1 to 10, where 1 = self-esteem is poor and 10 = self-esteem is excellent.

| | |
|---|---|
| 1 Self-esteem at work | 1 2 3 4 5 6 7 8 9 10 |
| 2 Self-esteem in your social life | 1 2 3 4 5 6 7 8 9 10 |
| 3 Self-esteem with strangers | 1 2 3 4 5 6 7 8 9 10 |
| 4 Self-esteem in your domestic/home life | 1 2 3 4 5 6 7 8 9 10 |

5  Self-esteem with a partner, spouse or
   closest friend                              1 2 3 4 5 6 7 8 9 10
6  Self-esteem with your family (of origin)    1 2 3 4 5 6 7 8 9 10
7  Self-esteem in emotional intimacy
   (for example, telling someone close
   that you are angry with them)               1 2 3 4 5 6 7 8 9 10
8  Self-esteem in sexual intimacy              1 2 3 4 5 6 7 8 9 10
9  Self-esteem about your appearance           1 2 3 4 5 6 7 8 9 10
10 Self-esteem about your personality          1 2 3 4 5 6 7 8 9 10

How comfortable are you with:

11 Expressing angry feelings (such as
   rage and frustration)                       1 2 3 4 5 6 7 8 9 10
12 Expressing other feelings (such as
   grief, sadness, joy)                        1 2 3 4 5 6 7 8 9 10
13 Dealing with criticism from others          1 2 3 4 5 6 7 8 9 10
14 Dealing with compliments from others        1 2 3 4 5 6 7 8 9 10
15 Dealing with perfectionism                  1 2 3 4 5 6 7 8 9 10
16 The best my self-esteem has been in
   the past month is:                          1 2 3 4 5 6 7 8 9 10

When? ..................................................................................

This was because ...............................................................

17 The worst my self-esteem has been in
   the past month is:                          1 2 3 4 5 6 7 8 9 10

When? ..................................................................................

This was because ...............................................................

18 I feel that my overall rating for self-
   esteem today is probably:                   1 2 3 4 5 6 7 8 9 10

## Using the ratings chart for further exploration

Review your chart and mark a little arrow under each rating to show whether that area has been getting worse or improving in recent weeks or months. For example, if you feel that your ability to express anger is getting slightly better, mark:

1 2 3 4 5 6 ⑦ 8 9 10

→

Likewise, if you think that it has been getting worse, you might mark:

1 ② 3 4 5 6 7 8 9 10

←

Use your journal to explore *when* and *why* things have been getting worse or better. What has changed in your circumstances that you see a deterioration or improvement in this life-area? What feelings and thoughts are different about this situation? What are you *doing differently* to bring about a deterioration (or improvement)? The chart will help you to find out which situations have *always* been difficult and which ones have only *recently* become difficult.

David, for example, noticed that his self-esteem when relating to his parents had deteriorated in the last few months. Before this time, he might have rated himself as '8' on the scale, feeling open and comfortable with his parents, whereas now it was more like '2'. David could find no obvious explanation for feeling tense and withdrawn with his mum and dad and had become depressed about it.

When I asked David to explore in more detail what had changed recently to bring about this radical drop, he realized that it was something to do with turning 30 years of age. Suddenly a penny dropped for David and he could see that he was making comparisons with his father at the same age. His father had become a successful businessman by the time he was 30, owning several well-located properties, which meant that he could semi-retire. David had subconsciously held on to the idea that when he reached this same milestone, he too should have created some major achievement. While his father had not mentioned his own success for many years, every time David had contact with him after his 30th birthday, he felt awkward and ashamed. He felt that his parents avoided any mention of how disappointed they must be that he had not reached the same level of achievement as his father at the same age.

Once David understood the *reasons* behind his drop in self-esteem in this area of his life he felt relieved. It gave him a positive impetus to question his own unrealistic expectations (his father had received a large legacy in his twenties), and was even able to discuss his shame with his parents. After a short period of time, David was able to rate his self-esteem when dealing with his family as higher than ever before, at '9', because of the understanding and honesty they were now all sharing.

### Exercise 14: Exploring your low ratings

If you scored below '5' on the ratings chart for any life-area, use your journal to reflect on the following:

- Why do I find this situation so difficult?
- What is really going on?
- What factors about my own history might be influencing this difficulty?
- What or who is holding me back in this area of my life?
- What do I fear most in this situation?
- How do I want to be in this area of my life?
- What would I be doing differently to score a '10'?

Through exploration of this kind you are likely to gain a clearer sense of the nature and level of your self-esteem and which areas in your life need the most attention. You will have developed your self-awareness by doing this exercise and hopefully gained some clarity and insight into where you need to move forward. You will also have separated your life into different areas, showing how self-esteem affects each part. In this way you may see that low self-esteem is not one blanket experience that covers every area of your life equally. In the next section we break down self-esteem even further.

## The elements of self-esteem

A lack of self-esteem can often feel like one big block in our lives. Other people seem to have lots of it and we seem to have none. There are in fact many facets to self-esteem and when we break it down into separate elements it is easier to tackle and less overwhelming. We can then focus on small steps to achieving improved self-esteem, rather than having to make a complete shift in our approach to life all at once. We may also find that there are some aspects of self-esteem that we feel better about than others. Take a look at the list of the elements of self-esteem below:

- Self-awareness (knowing *how* you feel and behave).
- Self-knowledge (knowing *why* you feel and behave in certain ways).
- Self-acceptance (being comfortable with your character, personality and physical appearance – understanding and loving yourself in spite of your flaws).
- Having self-worth (believing that you have value just as you are).
- Self-reliance (acknowledging your power, but also being able to ask for help).
- Assertiveness (standing up for what you want and need, showing respect for yourself and others).
- A sense of capability (knowing you can handle situations).
- Confidence (knowing and trusting your skills).
- A sense of purpose (knowing you contribute and have value and worth).
- Able to take responsibility (taking the lead or initiative, when appropriate).
- Able to be accountable (being able to manage the consequences of your actions, being answerable).
- Feeling a sense of security and stability (inner calm, contentment, trusting yourself).
- Feeling a sense of belonging (feeling a part of groups or society).
- Integrity (having values you believe in and act on).
- Able to see and explore choices and make decisions.
- Having coping skills and strategies (for stress, disappointment, frustration and so on).
- Having resilience (to setbacks and failings).

- Ability to problem-solve (to stand back from problems and not be overwhelmed by them, to take things step by step, to look at possibilities, and analyse objectively).
- Able to relate and connect to others (ability to listen, understand, engage, share, show compassion, share emotional intimacy and so on).
- Able to receive compliments.
- Able to let go of constant comparisons with others.
- Able to activate positive self-talk (to be able to access a nurturing inner-voice explored in Chapter 6).

(This is not an exhaustive list and you may be able to think of more elements of self-esteem which apply particularly to you.)

### Exercise 15: Exploring the elements of self-esteem

1 As you go through the list above, mark a tick at the side of the elements you believe you already possess, and an asterisk against the ones where you want improvement. This will help you to recognize those areas of self-esteem that are working and those that could be developed. Elements such as self-awareness, assertiveness, exploring choices, making decisions, developing coping skills and problem-solving are all skills that can be learnt.

   It is uplifting to realize that self-esteem is not something elusive that we are randomly blessed with, but something that can be systematically learnt in the same way that we might learn any other skill. While many self-esteem elements are covered in this book, you can find out more from books devoted exclusively to the separate elements (see Suggested reading at the end of this book). Furthermore, many major towns which run adult education classes are likely to have courses in assertiveness, managing stress (for coping skills), managing change (for resilience) or even meditation (for self-awareness), which will give you the opportunity to develop these individual elements of self-esteem. Another encouraging factor is that most of the elements in the above list have a knock-on effect on each other, so that when you start to improve in just one aspect, other elements of self-esteem improve too.

2 Apart from books, magazines and classes, there are often television programmes that can help you to build some of the individual elements of self-esteem. Series such as those where people have

improved their communication skills, have become more confident at meeting members of the opposite sex or learnt to dress to enhance their physical attributes can provide useful tips. You might also look around you for someone you know who seems to have developed the element of self-esteem you wish to improve. Instead of avoiding these people you could see them as a role model and learn from them. What do they do to be successful at the self-esteem element you are working on? Could you even talk to them about it?

## The self-esteem cycle

Another way of looking at self-esteem is to explore the *process* that produces an experience of either low or high self-esteem. Take a look at Figures 1 and 2, which show three distinct stages in determining self-esteem.

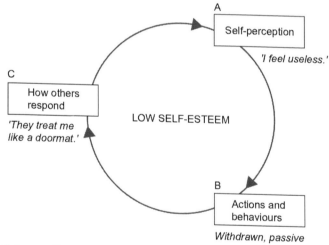

**Figure 1 Low self-esteem**

If you start at point A in the cycle with low self-esteem (Figure 1), you might be feeling (and saying to yourself) that you are 'useless'. The actions and behaviours that follow from this state of mind will be directly affected by this self-perception and you are likely to behave in a withdrawn manner (B). You may find, for example, that you do not engage with others and have nothing to say (because you believe it would be worthless). The result is at C – most people are likely to respond to your passive behaviours by ignoring you, not taking you seriously or putting you down. This in turn leads you to feel useless and inadequate again and you are back at square one, ready to repeat the same cycle in your next situation.

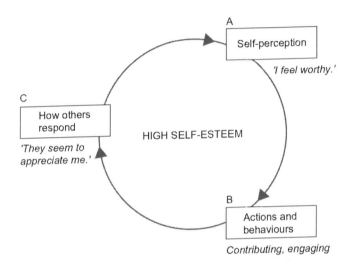

**Figure 2 High self-esteem**

Now look at another scenario (Figure 2). Imagine what the cycle would look like if you started out feeling positive and worthwhile about yourself (A). Your behaviours would follow through with this feeling so that you become involved and participate (B). The result is that others are likely to notice you and respond with respect and appreciation (C) and this gives you a feeling of being worthy, which takes you back to the starting point.

### Breaking the low self-esteem cycle

If you make positive changes *at any stage* in the cycle, it can have a profound effect on your self-esteem. If, for example, you were to develop your inner nurturing voice and feel more worthwhile (A), you are likely to feel you have more to offer (B) and therefore create more involvement and intimacy with others (C).

Making a change at (B) in the cycle, however, is the easiest change to make. If you can change your *behaviours*, even if only slightly, you are likely to see a positive cycle of events occurring. If you learn to act more assertively, people are likely to treat you with respect (C), and you will feel better about yourself (A).

Here is an example from Nicki's journal:

**Nicki, trainee designer, 22**

In meetings at work I used to die inside. I was so nervous and would not look up when I had to speak. I could not understand why people did not take me seriously; they often talked over me and ignored me. When I changed the tone of my voice, took my time and made proper eye contact (B), I received a different reaction – they really took notice of me (C). Then I felt like what I said was important and I felt more confident, like I really belonged to the team (A).

## Exercise 16: Using the self-esteem cycle

1  Copy down the cycle above and add your own words to describe the experiences which apply to you at each of the three stages *when your self-esteem is at its worst.*

2  Now draw the cycle again and put down at each point how you would *like to be, at your very best.* What would you feel about yourself at (A), how would you behave (B) and how might others respond to you (C)?

3  Think back. Have you ever felt self-esteem as good as your description in your response to question 2 above? What were the stages of the cycle then? If you cannot find an example of good self-esteem, can you find one when your self-esteem was just a little better than it is now? Could this be achieved again? What would you have to do differently at (B) in the cycle to improve your self-esteem?

4  Remember that stage (B) is the key to making changes. Your behaviour is a learnt habit and you can change your habits. Being more assertive, for example, is one of the first behaviours that can make a difference to your self-esteem.

In the next chapter we will explore how your upbringing has influenced your self-esteem and how you can challenge patterns of low self-esteem which may have been established in the family.

# 9

# Self-esteem in the family

## Your history of self-esteem

A useful way of shedding light on your own levels of self-esteem is to look at the history and patterns of self-esteem within your family as you grew up. Use your journal to answer the following questions.

### Exercise 17: Self-esteem in your family

1 Reflect on how being with your *father* (or father-figure) made you feel about yourself when you were growing up. Choose one or two of the words listed below (or find your own description), to sum up how you felt about yourself, when you were around your father, as a child:

> happy, sad, bad, angry, confused, misunderstood, safe, silly, neglected, inadequate, overlooked, quiet, special, clever, strong, weak, guilty, clumsy, difficult, small, childish, dull, boring, exciting, insignificant, sweet, ridiculed, unprotected, nervous, self-doubting, stupid (or use your own words)

My chosen words are: .................................................................. .

2 How did being with your *mother* (or mother-figure) make you feel about yourself when you were growing up? (Refer to the list above.)

My chosen words are: .................................................................. .

3 How would you describe the level of self-esteem felt and expressed by your father? How confident was he, in your eyes, as you were growing up? How did he show his self-esteem? What factors seemed to contribute to your father's level of self-esteem? (If your father was not present, how did family members who knew him portray his self-esteem?)

4 How do you regard his self-esteem now that he is older?

5 How would you describe the level of self-esteem felt and expressed by your mother? How confident was she, in your eyes, as you were growing up? How did she show her self-esteem? What factors seemed to contribute to your mother's level of self-esteem? (If your mother was not present, how did family members who knew her portray her self-esteem?)

6 How do you regard her self-esteem now that she is older?

7 What connections do you see between what you have written about your parents and your own self-esteem?

8 Are there any clues here as to why *your* self-esteem might not be as high as it could be?

9 Did you have brothers, sisters or any other family members who seem to have had a direct impact on your self-esteem? (For example, you may have been bullied or overprotected as a child, or been expected to carry too much responsibility.)

Belinda explained what she discovered when she did this exercise:

*Belinda, Spanish teacher, 35*
When I explored how I felt being around my father as a child, I realized it was mostly 'overlooked'. I didn't feel seen by my dad, or valued by him at all. He was either working or more interested in my two brothers. I realize now that he didn't treat my mum with much respect or interest either. Perhaps he felt that women were second-rate. I can see now where some of my low self-esteem could have come from, because I often defer to men and see them as more important. I definitely want to challenge this now and I certainly feel better about myself being able to see that there could be reasons for my low self-esteem in relationships.

When we understand some of the reasons why we might have developed low self-esteem, it can help us to see that it may not be entirely our fault. This is not so we can blame other people (such as our parents), but so we can realize that certain events and relationships from the past will have had an impact on us, even if there was never any harm intended. It may help us to develop more compassion for ourselves if we recognize that there may have been many reasons outside ourselves for our lack of self-esteem. If, knowing this, we can begin to stop blaming ourselves, this will increase our self-esteem. This is why understanding more about why we have the level of self-esteem we do is so important.

## Family scripts

There may have been a number of hidden factors in your family that have influenced your self-esteem. Most people carry around beliefs about themselves and the world that they may never name, but which influence their behaviours and the way they feel about themselves. Consider the following statements:

Life is a struggle.
If you're a girl, you won't be successful.
Children should be seen and not heard.
The world is basically full of evil.

These are some of the 'life-scripts' that have been carried around, often unspoken, in the families of clients I have worked with. Often people do not realize that a 'family script' has been influencing their lives. It is as though one of these negative beliefs becomes the foundation or 'blueprint' for the way a family operates. Family members get used to it, do not challenge it and so it perpetuates. Consider how different family morale might be if their life-script was one of the following:

Every cloud has a silver lining.
Life is what you make of it.
Everyone has his or her own unique talents.
The world is basically a good place.

### Where do life-scripts come from?

Life-scripts are usually based on a long-held attitude to life held by one or both parents. They might express a view about work, relationships, money, children, love, sex, religion and so on. Often a belief will be established by direct experience. During the world wars, for example, scarcity of food and other resources brought scripts such as 'Make do and mend' and 'Waste not want not' into being. Such beliefs are often passed on unchanged from generation to generation and may never be challenged.

A family script may be affecting your self-esteem without you realizing it. The significant issues for self-esteem are that the scripts originating from your family may either be out of date, or not applicable to you. You may be subconsciously living the script of one or both of your parents or grandparents and this may be blocking progress or success in your life.

## Exercise 18: Identifying life-scripts in your family

1 What do you think are (or were) your father's 'life-scripts' or sayings about life? Remember you may never have heard them spoken, but you might be able to pinpoint his beliefs from assessing his attitude to life. If you are not certain, make an intuitive guess.

2 What do you think are (or were) your mother's 'life-scripts' or sayings about life?

3 Are there any other family members who are likely to have influenced you? What were their 'life scripts'?

An excerpt from Jeremy's journal explains his insights around life-scripts:

### Jeremy, merchant banker, 41

When I explored the family scripts that seemed to have been around when I was growing up, I was quite shocked to realize they were so negative. My dad's life-script was definitely, 'Life will always be hard and you will never get anywhere.' My mum's was something like, 'I am a victim, I am weak.' Not a great recipe for good self-esteem for any of us! I realized that my own life-script was based on theirs and I did not want it to be. I could see that circumstances in both my parents' lives had led to them creating such negative scripts, but that these belonged to them and not to me. I had not experienced hardship in the same way they had and I could see hope and positivism in my outlook, which was different from theirs. I knew I needed to separate myself from my parents' script and find a more appropriate one of my own. I decided that my new life-script would be, 'Work hard and you will reap the rewards.' These simple words have changed my attitude to life completely. I now have more motivation and self-esteem, especially at work.

4 What is your view of life and the world? What do you think is your own life-script? Is it positive or negative? Is it someone else's script or is it truly your own? What are the likely life-scripts of people you admire? What would you *like* your life-script to be?

When you have found a life-script that you feel is positive and suits you, write it in a place where you will come across it from time to time to establish and reinforce it. Write it on a sticky note and attach it inside your appointments diary, your briefcase, handbag, sports locker or drawer.

## Distorted beliefs

Distorted beliefs can work in a similar way to life-scripts. We all create negative or positive beliefs from an early age about life and ourselves based on our experiences and the way others have reacted to us (see the section on inner self-talk explored in Chapter 5, pages 47–53). Negative self-beliefs associated with low self-esteem sound like the following: 'I am not good enough,' 'I am not lovable,' or 'I must change myself before I can be accepted.' These beliefs about ourselves are internalized and often labelled by us as 'the truth'. They may not, however, be true or valid.

During our upbringing, we may have misinterpreted or misconstrued events that led to negative self-beliefs being formed. As children we tend to take things at face value, and by not seeing the whole picture we may have internalized incorrect self-beliefs. We may not understand why someone important to us may have left the family, for example (through separation, divorce, illness or death). We may not see the hidden motives to explain why an adult may have behaved harshly or abusively to us. These reasons might be more obvious to an adult, but a child rarely questions what happens in the family or how he or she is treated. All the child experiences is the feeling of abandonment, rejection or fear and this can form the basis of a negative self-belief. A child might draw conclusions that it is because of him that parents have split up or that he is to blame for being abused. We do not realize that these beliefs are distorted and once they are established as part of us they seem to be set in stone. We then start believing them and acting as though they are true.

The extract below explains how Mel came to discover one of her long-held distorted beliefs. This belief, which felt like a truth, had played a major part in damaging her self-esteem:

*Mel, nutritionist, 38*
When I was seven and living in South Africa, my father organized a camping trip into the Bush. He took my older brother, but refused to take me so I was left behind. I'll never forget how abandoned I felt and from that day I internalized the belief that my father did not love me. Thirty years later, I reminded him of this incident, which had been so significant to me. He told me that it was because he loved me that he

couldn't risk taking me into the Bush. It was too dangerous and I was too small. He remembered his sadness at having to leave me behind. I've wasted 30 years of my life wondering why my father didn't love me enough. Finding out the truth has made a big shift in our relationship and I only wish I had asked him about it earlier.

## Exercise 19: Identifying distorted beliefs

1 Is it possible that you may have misinterpreted an event or situation, just as Mel did in the extract above? Can you think of an example of this?
2 Can you see that some of your beliefs about yourself might be distorted? What memories do you have about others' reactions to you that may have triggered a distorted belief?
3 Could you refer to the person or people involved and find out more information about what really happened?
4 Might the person at the source of the negative experience have been going through some problems (such as illness, depression, grief, mental instability) that might have caused them to behave in this way towards you? Might they have been unhappy about something which was unconnected to you?
5 List as many distorted beliefs as you can and begin to question them. You might like to refer to the tools for challenging statements and beliefs in Chapter 6 (page 54).

## Overpraise

Another kind of distortion can take place in families that could affect our self-esteem. It happens when one or both parents *overpraise* a child. This issue is rarely explored in literature about self-esteem, because on the surface it might seem to be a positive factor, but it is nevertheless significant. In her journal, Gita explained how she believed overpraise led to her low self-esteem:

*Gita, receptionist, 24*
My mum spent most of my childhood telling me how fantastic, clever and attractive I was. I felt very special as a child, particularly as I was the only child in the family. Everything I did was fussed over and I never seemed to put a foot wrong. You'd think this would lead to me having good self-esteem but in fact I think it caused the opposite. I expected everyone to see me how my mum did and of course this did not happen in the real world. If I was that clever, how come I didn't get

into university? If I was so special, how come I never had a boyfriend for longer than two months? By the time I was 18 lots of doubts had crept in. Maybe I wasn't that good after all? My self-esteem took a terrible knock as I realized that my mum's view of me was distorted and unreal.

It was only recently that I started to question what my mum was doing. Perhaps she wanted me to be a brilliant daughter so that she could feel she was being a good parent. Perhaps she was reacting to her own unhappy upbringing, by showering me with praise she never had. I believe my mother meant well, but she gave me a distorted belief about myself, which turned out to be damaging. I had to try to clear away the rose-tinted view my mum had projected on to me and realize that I was probably quite average at most things. This was hard to face at first, but now I know I have a realistic picture of myself and my abilities. I am able to aim for things I can achieve now, instead of constantly feeling like I am letting everyone down by aiming too high and failing. I have managed to build up my self-esteem in this way.

## Shoulds, musts and oughts

Further family influences on self-esteem come in the form of internalized 'shoulds, musts and oughts' which we all carry around with us. These are the 'rules' about how to behave which we have learnt from parents, teachers and other authority figures. Sometimes we will have clearly heard the 'shoulds, musts and oughts' over and over again. At other times we will have picked them up subconsciously:

You must never show your feelings.
You must get grade 'A's at school.
You're a girl, you should do needlework.
You're a boy, you should be athletic.

'Shoulds' messages are like the 'inner tape recordings' explored in Chapter 5 (page 47). They automatically start playing in our heads: 'You should invite your mother-in-law for Christmas,' 'You really ought to say you'll babysit for your sister,' 'You shouldn't help yourself to dessert until everyone else has had some,' and so on. Only when we bring these shoulds into the open, can we decide whether they are helping us or holding us back. If they are out of date or belong to someone else they are probably no longer necessary. First of all we need to use our self-awareness to identify which shoulds, musts and oughts play the biggest part in our lives. We can then assess how they might be inhibiting us and make choices about whether we still want to keep them. Instead of shoulds having control over us, we can then have some control over them.

## Exercise 20: Uncovering the 'shoulds, musts and oughts' in your life

1 The first step in challenging your shoulds is to become aware of the messages they contain. As you tune in to your inner self-talk, notice when one of them pops up, then stop and without judging yourself say,

'Oh yes – there's that "should" about being lazy again,' or 'There's that "must" about improving myself.' Write them down.
2 Do any of the shoulds on the list below sound familiar? Add the ones you identify with to your list:

I should be the perfect mother, friend, sister, lover, daughter, student, and so on.
I ought to be able to endure any hardship without needing help.
I must be cheerful and happy at all times.
I should be able to solve all my problems.
I should always be efficient and competent.
I should know, understand and foresee everything.
I should never have feelings such as anger, rage or jealousy.
I should never *show* feelings such as anger, rage or jealousy.
I must never make mistakes.
I should never change my mind.
I should never change my feelings about someone.
I should always be busy.
I should be totally independent and self-reliant.
I should never get tired or ill.
I should never be frightened or fearful.
I ought to be kind and generous all the time.
I must care for everyone who cares for me.
I should not take time merely for my own pleasure.
I must always be there for other people.
3 Add more shoulds to your list by reflecting on the following life-areas to see where you feel any recurring obligations, guilt or conflicts:

relationships, work, career, parenting, home life, creativity, sexual activities, politics, religion, money, self-image, addictions, food, health, fitness, expressing feelings

Guilt about something is a clue that there is a 'should' involved. For example, you might feel guilty for letting someone down because you carry a should saying: 'I should never put myself first.'

When you have a comprehensive list of shoulds, musts or oughts, choose the five most powerful ones and use your journal to complete the following exercise for each one.

### Exercise 21: Exploring 'shoulds'

1 Where did this 'should, must or ought' come from originally? Think back – do you remember who might have said or implied it?
2 How did this 'should' help you in the past? (For example, 'I must never make mistakes' might have helped you to be conscientious as a child.)
3 How does it help you now as an adult? Does it add value to your life? Does it hinder you?
4 Describe how you/your life would be, if you continued to obey this should.
5 Describe how you/your life would be, if you stopped obeying this should.
6 What are the drawbacks of obeying this should?
7 Do you want to keep this should? If not, how might you challenge it?

The above exercise allows you to examine your shoulds and see who they really belong to. If you no longer want or need a should you can challenge and change it. Try the following exercise with 'out-of-date' shoulds you want to be rid of:

### Exercise 22: Challenging and changing 'shoulds'

1  Take a few quiet moments on your own and imagine the person who 'gave' you this should. Picture them in your mind's eye as though they were with you now. In your imagination politely explain that you no longer need this should and would like to give it back to them. Imagine giving back a parcel or any other image that represents the unwanted should.

2  Change the wording of the should to make it more comfortable and reasonable. For example, 'I must never be lazy' might feel more acceptable if you said, 'I do not *want* to be lazy.' Rewrite your shoulds using terms such as 'I could', 'I'd like', 'I need' or 'I want' to 'soften' the shoulds and make them less absolute. In this way you are making your shoulds fit your life and not the other way around.

3  Reframe the should to make it more manageable and realistic. For example, 'I do not want to be lazy, but sometimes I need time to recuperate.' This allows you to see that shoulds need to be flexible and adapted to different circumstances.

You may need to return to this exercise if you have a long list of shoulds you wish to challenge. Large numbers of unrealistic shoulds probably mean that you are suffering from low self-esteem, because you are constantly trying and inevitably failing to live up to idealistic standards (usually someone else's standards which do not fit who you are). Only when we realize that some of these shoulds are unrealistic and perfectionist do we see how they are holding us back.

Challenging, modifying and adapting shoulds helps to reduce the 'not good enough' feeling. If you can transform shoulds and keep instead 'reasonable guidelines' which enhance your life and strengthen your motivation, self-discipline and moral conscience, this can benefit your self-esteem. You will not be constantly falling short of the so-called standards that unachievable shoulds create. This leads on to another common trait of low self-esteem, perfectionism.

## Perfectionism

People with low self-esteem often have very exacting standards for themselves, but expect lower standards from other people. I often hear my clients say something like, 'It's OK for other people to be off work with illness, but it's not OK for me,' or 'I'm quite happy to listen to my friend's problems, but she would never want to listen to mine.'

Perfectionism is a trap, because no matter how hard we try it is impossible to be perfect. It is human to make mistakes, fall ill and have problems. With low self-esteem we might think we need higher standards than anyone else in order to feel worthwhile. Perfectionism is about *proving ourselves* – it is about trying to show through what we do that we are acceptable.

With perfectionism, we are trying to aim for unrealistic standards in order to feel better about ourselves and in the end it only leaves us feeling worse. Ajay's example below is a good illustration of the perfectionism trap.

Until recently, Ajay felt confident and appreciated in his job in advertising and could not understand why he suddenly found himself staying late, taking on too many projects, not asking anyone for help and taking work home at the weekends. One day he ended up crying at his desk and had to take time off work because he could no longer cope with the pressure he was under. When he measured himself using the ratings chart (Chapter 8, pages 70–1), he gave himself a '1' for 'self-esteem at work'.

I asked Ajay when this 'overworking' had started and he realized that there had been a quiet period at work when he had barely any work to do and thoughts of redundancy had started going through his mind. Ajay had panicked and put himself under tremendous pressure to prove that he was an indispensable employee in a desperate bid to avoid redundancy. He was trying to prove he was not only essential, but also a 'perfect' member of the team.

I helped Ajay to see how his perfectionism was self-defeating. On a continuum of working harder and harder there comes a point when a person cannot sustain the pressure and things start falling apart. The very thing Ajay wanted to prove to his employers – that he was valuable and made a great contribution – became under threat because he was trying too hard. He had now become the opposite – a liability – so his intentions had completely backfired.

Once Ajay understood what he had been doing, he immediately made some adjustments. He told his manager about his fears of redundancy and they both acknowledged how difficult this uncertainty was. They also agreed he needed to cut back his working hours straight away. Ajay realized that if he were made redundant it would not be the end of the world and that he would be able to find another job. Within only one week, Ajay felt back on top of things and his self-esteem at work was rapidly increasing.

### Exercise 23: Are you trying to be perfect?

You might like to use your journal to look at areas of perfectionism in your life. Review your own standards – are they realistic high standards or are you expecting perfection? Can you sustain the standards you have set yourself or are you heading for burnout? Do you set standards for yourself that you are constantly failing to achieve? Do you end up defeating yourself in the end? Do you expect more from yourself than you would from someone else? Would you expect the same level from your best friend? Are you constantly on a mission to prove something to yourself or anyone else? If so, what are you trying to prove?

Setting high standards is different from setting perfectionist ones. The former can be achieved with hard work and effort, the latter will never be achieved. Can you adjust your standards so that they are achievable? Can you allow yourself some human failings now and again? Can you treat yourself like a best friend and challenge some of the idealistic standards you set for yourself? Can you let yourself off the hook from time to time and still feel worthwhile? If you work at these areas, not only is your self-esteem likely to improve, but also your health and well-being.

In the next chapter you will be expanding your journal writing to include body-felt feelings, images, drawings and dreams.

# 10

# Taking the journal further

## Listening to your body to find your feelings

I often find myself carrying around a feeling which I call my 'yuck' feeling. I know now that this feeling is a signal for me that there is something bothering me which I have not yet acknowledged or named. By focusing inward, paying attention to places in my body and using the following guidelines, I usually reach a point when I can say: 'So *that's* what this is all about.' I then see with clarity, because I have reached something inside myself which I had previously not been able to get hold of. After that point I experience a sense of relief and acceptance. I know what I am dealing with and I can find ways to take special care of that feeling.

I recently experienced my 'yuck' feeling sending me a message that something was wrong and the process went something like this. I settled myself in a comfortable place with no interruptions and focused my awareness on my body. With my eyes shut I slowly took my attention from one part of my body to another trying to pick up any sense that a feeling might be hiding there. I asked myself: 'Is this where the "yuck" feeling is?' I discovered a particular sensitivity in my chest area, which seemed to be restricting my breathing. It felt a bit like how it is after I have been crying. It was as though I had been secretly crying about something, but this was hidden even from myself.

I continued to stay in contact with the feeling in my chest, breathing into the feeling, holding my focus there rather than moving away from it. My entire attention was on this feeling, which I could not yet name. As I stayed fully attuned to it, I realized there was something about 'loss' in there. It was as though this feeling was touching loss and grief. At this point I knew I had made a clear connection with something genuine going on inside me and with this clarity came release and relief. I then needed to cry, although at this stage I did not know the reason for this.

As I continued to stay in contact with and accept my tears and the feelings in my chest, a further recognition brought me more understanding. Several days previously in a flurry of spring-cleaning, I had come across some old love letters and had decided in a matter-of-fact fashion to throw them away. Feelings associated with that action had only now caught up with me. The letters still had emotional resonance for me and I had been completely unaware of this when I had so casually discarded them. My feelings reminded me that I had some unresolved feelings about that relationship. This was what the grief and loss was about.

By remaining in full contact and with a willingness to listen to the root cause of my disturbance, I had reached the feelings themselves and their origin. The vague 'yuck' feeling I started with had been fully listened to, named and experienced. In doing so I felt an immediate shift in my mood. I suddenly felt much better and a new feeling was there – a great relief, now that it all made sense.

Without endeavouring to find the root of the problem I would have been left stuck and powerless. I would have remained 'in the dark' feeling 'yuck'. Writing my findings down gave me further clarity and release. The irony of this process is that by fully accepting the original difficult feeling, it then changes into something better.

## Exercise 24: Listening to your body to find your feelings

In order to do this exercise you need a willingness to touch upon something unknown. At the starting point, you will not know where the feeling may take you. It resembles shining a torch into a dark cellar and this can feel scary. The experience I described above involved discomfort as I cried and became upset by the feelings welling up inside me. Within a short time, however, I was experiencing something quite different. I felt liberated and I was free of the 'yuck' feeling which was causing me to be miserable and restless.

Try these guidelines for using your body to investigate feelings which you cannot name. Useful starting points for this exercise are when you are feeling agitated, restless and miserable without knowing why.

1 Find a place where you can relax completely and be undisturbed.

2 Close your eyes and become aware of the different parts of your body, starting with your feet.

3 Slowly and gently scan your body with the unnamed feeling you are experiencing in your mind. Ask yourself 'Is this feeling associated with this part of my body?' Pay particular attention to your stomach, solar plexus, ribcage, chest, throat, neck and shoulders.

4 Try to stay in touch with the original uncomfortable feeling and when you sense a connection with a particular part of your body, stay focused on and around that area. Ask yourself questions like, 'What is this feeling *really* about?', 'What is hiding under this feeling?' and 'What is this part of my body trying to tell me?'

5 Keep staying in touch with the original feeling and allow your mind to associate with other feelings which might be connected. You will probably know when you have found a word which fits your feeling. It will somehow feel right and you will know that this is part of what the original feeling is about.

6 Keep doing this, peeling away layer after layer until you feel you have discovered every aspect of the feeling that you can for now.

7 Turn to your journal and write down all the feeling-words which seemed to resonate.

8 Explore these feeling-words further to see if you can gain any more information or understanding from them. Keep writing in an open, exploratory way and freely associate, allowing your mind to respond to and be guided by these feelings.

9 You will know that you have completed this process when you reach a point of clarity and release. The original feeling is likely to have shifted. If you do not reach this point, make an appointment with yourself to return to this feeling at some time in the near future.

This process can take some practice at first and you will need to trust that the feelings you have are there to help you to understand or to teach you something. The feelings will be there anyway, whether you acknowledge them or not and by not paying attention to them they may be causing you harm. They will be suppressed and will not have the chance to be healed or resolved.

In therapy, most people have a fear of digging deeply into their feelings, but it is my experience that the fear of what they might find is always worse than the feelings they actually discover. When you surrender to your feelings, not only are you respecting your feelings more, but you are taking care of your innermost emotional self. You will be learning to accept all of who you are. Such steps can only increase your self-esteem. By using your journal to label and record your feelings, you will be able to notice patterns, prepare yourself better for situations, anticipate your unique sensitivity to circumstances and discover what you need to do to look after those sensitivities.

You can find out more about this method by reading *Focusing* by Eugene Gendlin (see Suggested reading at the end of this book).

## Using images, symbols and metaphors

There may be times when you try to locate and name a feeling and it remains out of your reach. Or perhaps you are someone who tends to experience feelings in terms of images, symbols and metaphors. If so, you can use your journal to explore and understand your emotions through drawings, scribbles, word-pictures and diagrams. Joseph's example shows how he uses images in his mind to describe his depression:

### Joseph, plasterer, 23

I don't know what I am feeling exactly, but I feel black and gluey inside. It seems to be buried inside my stomach and is particularly bad at the end of the day. When I try to get close to it, it seems to want to destroy me, it seems angry with me – like it wants to drown me in the sticky tar.

Tanya shows how she explored her feelings about the termination of her pregnancy using shapes and words (page 95).

Both Joseph and Tanya were able to reach deeper feelings by allowing the images and symbols which represented their pain to unfold. Images, symbols and metaphors are wonderful tools to use for exploration. They help us to see our situation in a different way and make feelings more concrete. Images also seem connected with our subconscious and dreamworld. Working with them allows us to access useful insights which may have eluded us if we had stayed only on the level of using words.

I feel like this inside

It's like knives /// there's
a wound and blood ;' like
my heart is bleeding
and crying - this
is <u>hurt</u>.

I am broken with
hurt.
My heart is broken.
A pool of sadness.

I know what it is now. This is my pain and guilt. Yesterday
was the anniversary of my Termination. I can stay with this
for a few moments I can hold this pain and guilt I can
still love myself.
                                            Tanya

**Tanya, photographer, 26**

## Free-drawing in your journal

Here are some ideas for exploring your feelings through image-work: You can do 'free-drawing' at any time, but like the 'agony aunt' method (see Chapter 4, page 29), first thing in the morning, even sitting in bed before you do anything else, is a good time. The reason for this is that you have not yet moved into your daily routine and you are still in a half-dreamy state, which will allow subconscious images to arise more easily. Like the 'agony aunt' process, this is a clearing process to help you to express feelings you may not know are there.

### What is 'free-drawing'?

This is not an exercise in artistic ability, but is instead about bringing forward ideas, images, patterns, information, and hidden feelings in symbolic form, directly from the subconscious, without using any intellectual or rational input.

### Exercise 25: Free-drawing

To do a 'free-drawing', you need a blank sheet of paper and you start moving your chosen crayon, pen or paint-brush straight away *without thinking or directing*. It is fundamental in this kind of work to draw directly from your intuition and to allow the drawing materials to take you where they want to go. You may end up with an entirely abstract picture as a result, or something with familiar shapes in it. Either way is fine, as long as it feels undirected by any premeditation. This time, instead of asking yourself 'How am I feeling?' – just start moving your crayon.

When you have completed your drawing, you can explore your ideas and shapes using the following three stages, making notes as you go along. Only refer to these stages *after* you have completed your drawing and try to empty your mind of the criteria when you do your next drawing, so that you are not influencing your picture. Be aware that in the initial stages of exploration, you are only noticing and observing what is there in your picture and how you drew it. Interpretations come later.

*Stage 1: Exploration*
Ask yourself the following questions. The responses in italics refer to Janet's free-drawing (see page 97).

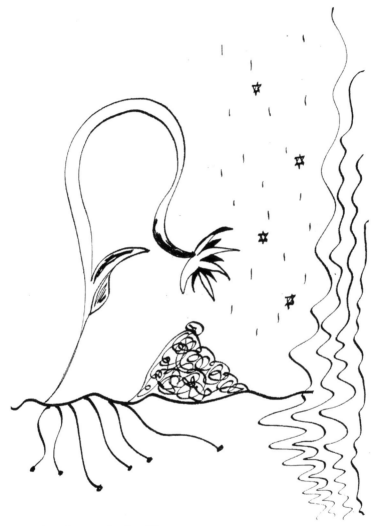

**Janet, hotel receptionist, 37**

1 When you look at the completed picture, what are your overall impressions? *It seems to be about growth.*
2 How would you describe the style of the picture? *It is flowing, with no rough edges.*
3 What colours have you used and which ones dominate? *All the colours are earthy ones – browns and greens.*

4 How was your use of space? *It feels unbalanced and part of it seems off the page.*

5 What was the pace of the drawing as you drew it? *It speeded up towards the end, when I felt an urgency to fill in the right side quickly.*

6 What are the inter-relationships between different parts of the picture? *There are three main areas and they seem connected.*

*Stage 2: Free association*

1 Now freely associate with this picture. What do the elements in it remind you of? Are there any hidden memories here? Are there any insights or intuitive connections to other aspects of your life? (Janet's response was: *The colours are basic to nature: greens, browns and blues. It seems to be about the real essence of life.*)

2 Now suggest a few possible titles for the picture, as though you are looking for the story hidden there, like the title of a book or film (*Distorted Growth* or *The Rot has Set In*).

3 Find three key words which sum up the most significant aspects or connotations of this picture. Take your time over this. You might identify several words and then underline the three with most significance or emotional 'pull' to them (*striving, tired, precarious*).

4 How would the image need to be altered or changed in order for it to be resolved, healed or more balanced? What would need to happen in the picture for you to feel better about it? (*I want the flower to stand up tall and straight. I want the pile of mud to disappear.*)

*Stage 3: Interpretation*

1 Finally, use the picture as a metaphor and 'map' it back on to your life at the moment, by asking yourself:

> What is this picture telling me about me or my life right now?
> What information does this picture have for me?
> What can I learn about myself right now from this picture?
> What does this mean to me?
> What is the best thing which is emerging from this exploration?
> What is the worst thing?

2 What new step might you need to take as a result of the messages that this image is conveying to you?

3 Where might things end up if you *do not* make any changes? What would happen to the image? What would happen to your life?

Remember that the image may represent only a part, not all of you or your life. For example, the picture may reflect your underlying feelings about your career, your relationships or sense of purpose, and so on. Whichever area you feel the image is referring to is the area your subconscious wants you to focus on at this present time.

Janet shares her interpretation of her free-drawing (see page 97):

*Janet, hotel receptionist, 37*
From this picture I see that my growth seems to have dried up. The plant is buckled and rotting and I can feel how very tired I am. I have nothing more to give. Like the plant, I need basics like water and sunshine. I need to walk by the river and sit on a beach somewhere. I feel burnt out and I didn't realize how much, until I drew this picture! It makes me feel sad to see this poor bending flower that is actually me, but I also feel determined to do something about it.

When you do a series of free-drawings, date them and then look for links with your previous pictures.

Janet made this journal entry after completing several free-drawings:

I see the theme of growth emerging in all my pictures so far, and I can see how essential this aspect of my life is for me. I know this is what I want – to be growing, learning and moving on. Previously, I felt I'd got to a point in my life when I couldn't find any more dreams I wanted to achieve. Now I can see that there is more growth to come and I want to find inspiration and adventure in my life once more.

## Using image-work without drawing

If you do not wish to draw or feel unable to put your images on the page, here are some alternative ideas for exploring your feelings through image-work.

### Exercise 26: Working with images in your mind

1 Try to find an image in your mind for your feelings or for the situation you find yourself in. You may, for example, feel 'trapped in a box' or feel like the 'world is closing in on you'. Try to describe any shapes and pictures which come to mind. Sketch them on paper if you can, if not, just explore the images as they present themselves in your mind's eye.

2 What feelings do you associate with the shapes in your image-description? What story do the shapes tell?

3 Where is this image? Is it located inside your body? Does it remind you of anything? Imagine the image in front of you projected on to

a large cinema screen. What else is near, behind or above the image when you see the bigger picture? What else is in the background?

4  Imagine stepping into the image on the screen. What happens if you try to step alongside the image? What feelings arise for you as you remain close by this image?

5  What happens if you try to step into the shape itself? Can you become the image? How does that feel?

6  Be an observer to this image again. Where does the shape or image want to go to next? What is the next natural step for this image? Is it unfolding into another image? Is something else emerging?

7  Ask the image what it is trying to tell you. Ask what message it has for you. Ask what it needs from you.

8  What would have to happen to the image for an improvement or progress to take place? Can you allow this to unfold? How does this affect the feelings you associate with this image?

9  What would the image have to do to be resolved or be at peace? How does this relate to the associated feelings you have?

By working on the images which represent the feelings, we are also working with the feelings themselves. You may now be in a position to write in your journal about this exercise. Dina Gloubermann's excellent book *Life Choices, Life Changes* will give you more ideas if you like this method (see Suggested reading). The combination of drawing and writing can help you see an overview of your journey during this stage of your life. You might also record what you learnt from your drawings, such as what you need and where you are heading.

## The dream journal

Our dreams are a useful source of wisdom to us. Dreams emerge from our subconscious and often contain 'messages' for us, which we are not yet aware of in our waking life. By keeping a record of your dreams you can look for any messages your subconscious is trying to convey to you. Recurring dreams are usually linked to some issue which is unresolved and the same themes may appear in your dreams until the issue is identified and dealt with.

In order to keep a dream journal, you need to keep your book beside your bed and write in it the very instant that you wake from a dream. If you decide to make a cup of tea or get the slightest bit distracted, the dream will dissipate in a matter of moments. Write down as much of the dream as you can remember in the order it seemed to happen. The more detail you include, the more chance you have of noticing recurring patterns. Note how you *felt* in the dream as well as the events which occurred.

When you have recalled all you can, give the dream a title to convey the essential focus of the dream, something like 'Getting out of the storm' or 'Being angry with Jack'. Underline any key words which invoke a powerful feeling or which seem significant. Then set your dream journal aside for the next night.

The messages in dreams often emerge over the period of a few weeks. As you build up your collection of dreams, look back to earlier ones to compare the titles and the key words. See if any themes or patterns emerge. Ask yourself what these themes mean to your waking life and what would have to change or be resolved for the dreams to move on. Sometimes this can involve facing up to an issue you have been avoiding or denying.

Marianne made a surprising discovery when she began to record her dreams:

*Marianne, actress, 29*
I started to realize that my dreams were connected to accommodation of different sorts. In one dream there would be a cottage I was moving into, next a hall of residence at college, next some campsite in the middle of nowhere. When I explored the feelings that were present, I saw that in each dream I felt pushed out – it wasn't my home or I wasn't welcome. Sometimes other people's clothes were in the cupboards or my key wouldn't unlock the front door.

So then I looked at my waking life to see what message these dreams were trying to tell me. It suddenly struck me that I was not comfortable around my flatmate at home. What is weird is that I had not realized this at all on a conscious level! As soon as I saw the significance of the dreams, I noticed how being there didn't feel like my place any more. I felt awkward around her and saw how we didn't really get on. I then realized that we needed to have an honest talk about it. The next month she moved out. I felt much happier and I stopped having those kinds of dreams.

By keeping a dream journal you may find that you remember your dreams more often and you will therefore have a powerful source of information to guide you. In Chapter 11 we look at creating useful shorthand 'maps' in the journal.

# 11

# Getting clearer

This chapter invites you to try some shorthand journal writing using 'maps'.

## Mind-maps

We have already looked at exploring thoughts and feelings and one easy method of taking this further is to use a 'mind-map'. Mind-maps are a shorthand way of searching for clarity. They are useful when you are too muddled or anxious to write down your thoughts in sentences or do not have the time to do so. Because mind-maps are not linear, you can add to the page without being concerned about the order of your ideas or how they might fit together. You can also add to a mind-map over a period of days.

### Exercise 27: Creating a mind-map

1 To start a simple mind-map you need to have some idea of what you want to focus on. Put down any word or phrase that you want to explore in the centre of your sheet. It could be 'depression' or 'my life right now' or it could be a person's name, an event, something you are struggling with or any other topic you wish to write more about.

2 Then start adding some of the predominant feelings, thoughts, memories and ideas you are experiencing in connection with your central focus. It might look something like Map 1 on page 103.

3 Keep brainstorming and adding words, even if they seem unconnected to your original topic, and allow yourself to do this quickly without thinking about it too much.

4 When you seem to have run out of words, take a look at the whole pattern and see if there are any links or if certain words are related to each other. If so, find a way of showing the connections, using circles, boxes, arrows or any other marks.

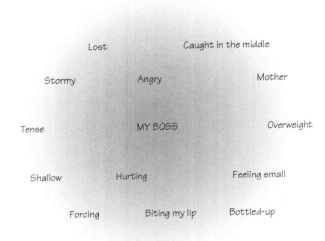

**Map 1**

5  Next, think of a title for your map, a phrase which sums up what this issue is all about (see Map 2, page 104).

Mind-maps build on free association – the process of allowing one word or idea to quickly leap to another one without too much 'thinking' being involved. You may find that your subconscious mind brings forward ideas that you had not yet known were connected. At this point you may feel the urge to write things out in more detail, or to question why certain thoughts have emerged. Seeing some connections or new ideas may be enough for you to move forward with your issue. Hopefully by undertaking this process you will at least have more clarity about the subject itself. From this point you may want to draw up some action points for dealing with your situation better.

If you wish to take mind-maps further, try the worry map idea overleaf.

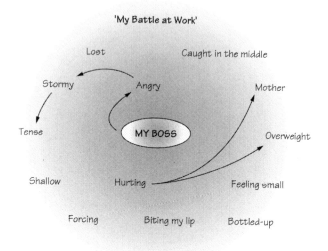

'My Battle at Work'

Lost  Caught in the middle

Stormy  Angry  Mother

Tense  MY BOSS  Overweight

Shallow  Hurting  Feeling small

Forcing  Biting my lip  Bottled-up

**Map 2**

## Creating a worry map

One powerful way of dealing with worry and anxiety is to create a 'worry map'. This technique invites you to work through the 'agony aunt' method, the 'four constructive tasks' and the 'problem-solving' process described in Chapter 4. The easiest way to demonstrate the process is by using a genuine example, taken from work with a client in counselling.

### Case history: Alan's worry map

Alan was a 40-year-old client who was feeling completely overwhelmed. He felt he had so much going wrong in his life, and so much internal upheaval that he could not cope any more. He felt he was in a complete mess and was suffering from low self-esteem. During the session, I asked him to try to identify as many parts of this 'mess' as he possibly could so I could write them down. Our conversation went something like this:

## 1 The 'agony aunt' method (emotional level)

*Alan*: I don't know where to start – it is all so big and tangled up ...

*Alison*: I can see you're on the verge of going under with all this confusion. Just start anywhere you can with the first thing on your mind and I will write your worries down, as you tell them to me. We can try to put them in some kind of order later. Let's just try to get them all out into the open first ... (I am encouraging Alan to express himself using the 'agony aunt' method from a purely feelings-based perspective. The only difference is that I am doing the writing.)

*Alan*: Well, one thing is this real rage I get into with Ruby, my girl-friend. She can be so cutting with me and it really makes my blood boil. Then there's the fact that we are living with her mother at the moment and Ruby always takes sides against me. I get angry with myself for not being able to cope with it. Then my father died in June and I don't think I've dealt with it properly ...

*Alison*: Go on ... (As Alan speaks *I* am putting each concern in a separate circle on the page.)

*Alan*: Yeah, there is a lot of stuff going on around my father ... childhood things which have been coming back ... the way he left when I was 12 ... all the rows he had with my mother ...

As Alan continued, I used the page to make a 'map' of worries. When he seemed to have mentioned everything for the time being, I showed him the map for his comments. The first thing he said was, 'I can't believe this is all there is ...', and he expressed relief and surprise that all his problems seemed to be there, but they were all contained within one page. His fantasy was that there were thousands of problems and that if he started to list them, he would go on for ever.

## 2 The 'four constructive tasks' (cognitive level)

I then asked Alan to consider the four constructive tasks (outlined in Chapter 4). He began to look for themes and patterns and to draw lines between the circles where there were links. He could see that the problems were not all random, but that they fell into broader themes (such as all the things which were making him 'angry' and all the issues which were to do with 'loss'). I also asked Alan to identify those issues which were uppermost in his mind and those which could be put on hold for a while. He then numbered the issues according to their importance, the most urgent one being his relationship with his girlfriend, Ruby.

Alan used ideas from the map to get an overview of his life at that time. Alan realized that the rage he had been feeling towards Ruby was probably more like 'hurt' for not feeling appreciated enough. He identified too that many of his current feelings reminded him of his childhood and in particular of feeling afraid and insecure as a young child. Alan summarized this present period of his life by calling it 'Feeling Powerless'. He was now using his thinking and analysing skills to explore the issues before him. He took the sheet away to think more about it and to add to it when he discovered new related issues.

Map 3 on page 107 shows how Alan's worry map looked at this stage.

### 3 The 'problem-solving' process (action level)

Following the steps of the 'problem-solving' process in Chapter 4, Alan went on to mark the areas where he felt he had some control and those areas where he felt he did not. This allowed him to see that there were areas where he had more choice than he thought and where he could take some action to improve the situation. Even in the areas where he did not have obvious control (for example, the way Ruby was treating him), he saw that there were steps he could take to feel better (such as finding ways to explain how hurt he felt at a time when Ruby was calm and receptive to listening to him).

Starting with Alan's most urgent issue, I asked him to identify any possible courses of action he could take to tackle his problems. We looked at similar situations from his past and how he had managed these. He evaluated how useful previous problem-solving techniques would be to him now and also looked at entirely new possibilities. Alan explored, for example, how he might include Ruby's mother in more of their social activities, and the actual words he might use to address his hurt with Ruby.

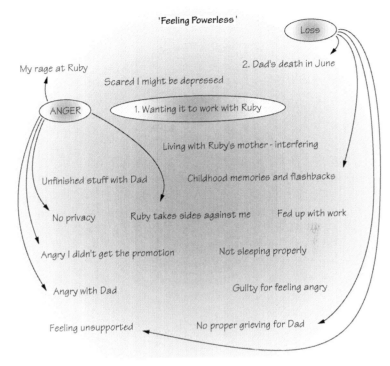

**Map 3**

We then broke these ideas down into smaller manageable stages. Alan made a list of the very first steps he could take towards putting these changes into practice and was able to draw up a list of small tasks which looked like this:

| Task | When |
|---|---|
| 1 Decide on a good time to talk to Ruby. | This evening when she is relaxed after her bath. |
| 2 Get hold of details of the opera. | Get listings magazine at news agent tonight. |
| 3 Discuss it with Ruby first and then invite her mother to an opera. | Maybe tonight if Ruby agrees. |

By the following session, Alan came in looking much brighter:

I felt such relief after the last session, as though a great burden had been lifted. I see that I can do something about my situation – I had felt so powerless and overwhelmed before.

Shifting worries out of our heads and on to a sheet of paper can be powerful. Once on paper, we can see the following:

1 There may not be as many concerns as we thought.
2 The worries usually appear more manageable.
3 Links and patterns become more obvious. This means that worries can often be broken down into far fewer main areas to be worked on, rather than hundreds of unconnected difficulties.
4 Once the worries are 'out there', we may feel that the time is right to start doing something about them. When they stay whirring around in our heads, we often play and replay the same old 'worry tape', but nothing changes.
5 Once everything is on the page, concerns can be prioritized, so that it does not feel as though everything has to be dealt with at once. Some issues will feel urgent while others can be put on hold for a while.
6 Our self-esteem tends to improve once we feel we are more in control.

After working through this process, Alan was much clearer about how his situation could be improved. The small action points meant that he could start to put these changes into immediate effect.

You can create your own worry map by following the stages above in conjunction with Chapter 4.

## The self-esteem wish-map

This creative and colourful exercise helps you to establish a future vision for yourself with more self-esteem. A sense of where we are heading in our lives gives us a focus of energy. When we are clear about the *outcomes* we want, it is easier to concentrate our efforts towards those goals. Once goals are clearly mapped out on the horizon, all we need to do is more things which take us closer to them and less things which do not. Furthermore, when we do not have a clear focus of where we are heading, we might spend long periods of time drifting or hoping for things to get better, without knowing what 'better' would consist of.

Whenever we set up the intention to do something positive, that is where our energy will be, even on a subconscious level. Our mind registers the desire (if it really is what we truly want), and then we will notice and create opportunities in line with this desire. Once you identify a genuine focus, energy towards it will be activated.

### Exercise 28: Creating your self-esteem wish-map

You can create a wish-map for one or several goals in your life (such as fitness, health, where you want to live, the job you would like to do and so on), but here we will concentrate on a wish-map for improving self-esteem.

1 Start with some crayons, a sheet of paper or card, a range of different magazines and some scissors. Look through the pages of each magazine and cut out anything which attracts your eye in connection with how you want to feel about yourself. It might be a picture of someone looking confident or a bowl of fruit which represents your wish to eat more healthily. Cut out anything which appeals to you or seems significant to improving your self-esteem. Then stick these cuttings on to a fresh sheet of paper or card.

2 If you are not exactly sure which factors would be part of your life with better self-esteem, cut out pictures which represent the feeling or experience you want to have. For example, one goal might be to feel 'calmer' or feel 'more in control' in your life. Find pictures which reflect these experiences for you (for example, a photo of someone doing yoga may convey the feeling of calm you are looking for).

3 Add anything extra to your picture using crayons to represent factors that you cannot find in your magazine. Use symbols, doodles or words to signify these other elements. Try to be as clear as you can about what you want. For example, instead of writing the word 'happiness', ask yourself what 'happiness' really means to you (such as 'adventure', 'feeling valued' or 'succeeding at college').

4 At the top of your finished map add the words: 'This is now my reality'. This statement establishes your intention to achieve your wish-map, but also allows your desires to come to you in a slightly different form to the one you might envisage.

5 Keep referring to your wish-map on a daily basis and focus on the good feelings you would experience on achieving it. This is where the motivational energy inside you begins to work and you are likely to find opportunities, coincidences, new ideas, or inspiration to move you towards your goal.

Louise described the benefits of doing her self-esteem wish-map:

*Louise, widow, 56*
I realized I had been too vague about some of the changes I wanted to see with regard to my self-esteem. I wanted to love myself more, but I couldn't break this down into anything concrete. When I did the wish-map, I came across some images in the magazines of how I wanted to feel. I cut out a picture of people laughing and a picture of children running free. This represented my desire to tackle my shyness in company and to really take care of the 'child part' of me.

I looked at my completed picture and felt how liberating it would be to have more self-esteem. I would be free from my terrible self-consciousness. One of the cuttings had people dancing and at first I thought, 'I want that feeling, but I'll never be able to do that.' The following week I noticed a poster in the local library advertising dance classes for the over-50s and I wrote down the contact number. I haven't rung up yet, but I know I have never been this close to joining some-thing like this on my own. I hope this time I'm going to get there.

In the final chapter we look at some quick journal techniques and how to review your journal to get the most out of it.

# 12
# Bringing it all together

## Quick journal tools

This chapter contains some quick but effective journal tools to use when you are short of time, plus some ideas to encourage you to use and review your journal regularly, to help you get the most out of it.

## The 'pillow book'

### Exercise 29: Creating a 'pillow book'

This is a delightful exercise and only takes two minutes at the end of each day. The exercise is to write just one statement about the day that you feel positive about. It could be something you did that you were pleased with or proud of, it could be something someone said to you, or something you noticed (such as a sunset or a butterfly). Ask yourself: 'What made me smile today?', 'What lifted my spirits today?', 'Which one moment do I want to cherish?'

The purpose of the pillow book is to create a collection of private uplifting memories. At the end of the year you will have a book full of positive moments which were all part of your personal experience. You can take a look at your book when you are feeling low and in need of a boost or when you want to remember the kinds of things you were doing and noticing during certain periods in your life. I have kept a pillow book beside my bed for at least four years. If you are like me and have a poor memory for day-to-day activities, it is invaluable as a reminder that you are present in each and every day and that there are little daily gems worth treasuring.

# Daily questions

If you do not have time to record your feelings in full in your journal, or time to reflect and explore, try to respond, every day, to just one of the questions in the following exercises:

### Exercise 30: At the beginning of the day ...

- What am I looking forward to today?
- What about today will fit the kind of life I aim to live?
- What will I do more of to build my self-esteem?
- What will I do less of to build my self-esteem?

### Exercise 31: At the end of the day ...

- What was better or working well today?
- On a scale of 1 to 10, where is my level of self-esteem or well-being today?
- What would have to happen for me to reach the next number on the scale?

# 'To-do' lists

### Exercise 32: Drawing up a 'to-do' list

This is a useful exercise when you are feeling overwhelmed with tasks. Use a sheet of paper divided into three columns. List all the things you can think of that need to be done, writing and numbering each task on a separate line. You might include only 'work' tasks, or it could be domestic chores or other specific tasks (such as planning for a holiday) or you can list *all* the tasks you know need to be done at the present time.

Then in the second column mark down approximately how long you think this particular task will take you – it might be five minutes or two hours. In the third column mark down the deadline by which time this task needs to be completed.

When you look at your entire list, check out what can be realistically achieved in one day. For example, if the anticipated time required for completing all your tasks totals 36 hours, with around 15 waking hours available in the day, much of your list will not be completed in 24 hours. Then look at your deadlines and decide which items must definitely be completed by the end of today. Can any tasks be broken down into smaller ones? If there are too many tasks for today, can you leave any of them until another day? What would be the worst that could happen if you did? Can you put back any of the deadlines? Who would you need to consult if you had to do this?

Then decide what you will set as your realistic target for today and what can be put off until tomorrow. Write these on a separate sheet or highlight them.

This exercise is useful for the following reasons:

- It helps you to see exactly what needs to be done. Sometimes we panic when there are lots of chores going around in our head. Once they are on paper, they can seem more manageable. You can also break big tasks down into smaller items to make them less daunting.
- We often forget that some tasks take a lot less time than we imagine. A list of ten items may look insurmountable, when in reality they might only take five minutes each. In under an hour you could have cleared these ten tasks from your 'to-do' list.
- When we get clearer about how long the tasks are likely to take and when they need to be completed, we start to feel more in control. When we feel more in control, our self-esteem increases, because we feel we can cope with the situation.

## Mood graphs

### Exercise 33: Learning from a mood graph

You can also use your journal to track particular cycles, such as the menstrual cycle or cycles at work. You could draw up a graph to show mood-swings or stress levels and fill this in on a daily basis to see any patterns. This helps you realize that certain states of mind may be linked to hormones, times of the month, the nature of your work, or other environmental factors such as pollen, air quality or daylight (as in Seasonal Affective Disorder, for example). By understanding connections in this way, you can see that your well-being is not random and you have the opportunity to prepare in advance for problematic stages in your particular cycle.

## The value of rereading your journal

One of the benefits of keeping a journal is that over a period of time you will have a record of your life and how you have dealt with situations. With the benefit of hindsight you can bring even more clarity to situations and consolidate your learning. You will be able to see the ways in which you have changed and the ways you have stayed the same. You will be clearer about your needs, values and goals. When you read back over your writing you can notice similar themes which keep cropping up. You can also recognize that feelings can pass – sometimes all they need is space and time.

Here are some exercises you can do as you read over previous journal entries:

### Exercise 34: Patterns

Look for patterns and repeated words. If you are in a problematic situation at the moment, do you remember being in similar situations before? Track them down in your journal and find out how you dealt with the difficulties before. What helped last time? What can you use again?

### Exercise 35: Themes

It is useful to put notes or mini stickers in the margin when you reread, so that you build in points of reference and can locate subjects and themes at a later stage. Maybe a section was about a struggle with money or how to be a parent. You can expand on these themes and describe what you have learnt from that stage in your life-journey. Then you will see the way in which your experiences are contributing to your development.

### Exercise 36: Turn things around

When you read about difficult or painful circumstances, ask yourself, 'What was the positive thing about this?' and 'How can I make sure this doesn't happen again?' In this way you are making use of your journal to see a bigger picture or a new perspective.

## Exercise 37: Pay-offs

When you continue to repeat behaviours which cause you pain, there has to be something positive you are getting out of it. Are you pursuing short-term gratification at the expense of long-term harm? This may be hard for you to accept, but there will be a 'pay-off' or gain for you if you are recreating the same kind of dysfunctional patterns in your life. The reason for the 'pay-off' may not be obvious, but it is likely to come from a deep emotional need or fear.

For example, an overweight person who continues to overeat, even though they hate this aspect of themselves, may secretly fear that if he or she were slim, there would no longer be an excuse for not having a romantic partner. As it stands, the person can tell themselves that a relationship is out of the question, because they secretly (or even subconsciously) hope their size makes them undesirable. This may stem from a deeply rooted fear of intimacy and their eating protects them from having to face this fear. Avoiding the fear of intimacy is the 'pay-off'.

- Are there any fears driving patterns of behaviour which are causing you distress?
- What are your pay-offs for repeating self-sabotaging behaviours?

## Exercise 38: The history of a problem

When you come across areas of difficulty in your life and especially if this difficulty recurs, trace a 'history' of this problem back to your upbringing. Your issue might be something concrete like money, careers or sex, or it could be a dynamic such as power, avoiding responsibility, guilt or betrayal. Travel back in time with these issues and look at how other members of your family dealt with them. Often we do not realize that a problem belongs not only to us, but also to others we grew up with, stemming from conditions within our family.

### Exercise 39: Create a resource

At times when you feel life is working well, or you feel you have higher self-esteem, ask yourself what you are doing differently to feel this way. Record the good habits you form, choices you make, beneficial strategies and what keeps you going. Then you will have a resource of methods which work well for you, which you can deliberately recreate. This is particularly helpful for difficult situations which recur in your life, such as stressful periods at work or life-transitions such as pregnancy. When you face these situations again, your journal will contain a ready-made plan of resources to help you.

### Exercise 40: Explore alternatives

When situations are uncomfortable, use your journal not only to write out your feelings, but to explore how you might respond differently. List the things you *could* do to empower yourself.

### Exercise 41: Review your boundaries

One way of feeling more empowered is to review your boundaries. Your boundaries are the unspoken rules you have when relating to other people. Boundaries provide your protection and create guidelines so that others know how you are to be treated. These hidden rules show what you will, and will not, tolerate from other people. They also involve how much you are prepared to offer people in terms of your time, availability, help, resources and so on.

Someone with unclear boundaries may allow people to use them or do things to them that are damaging or detrimental. For example, being able to say 'no' is a boundary issue. When you are clear in yourself about this boundary, other people know where they stand with you. If you are unclear, people may 'walk all over you', because they see that you 'cannot say no'.

Poor boundaries usually equate with low self-esteem, so to improve your self-esteem look for ways to tighten up your boundaries. Find issues connected with boundaries in your journal and list them. Note how you would like to change them so that you could avoid hurtful or problematic scenarios (it might be useful to think of someone you know who has 'good boundaries' and imagine what they would do).

### Exercise 42: Get back in control

One of the biggest boosts you can give to your self-esteem is to feel *in control*. This might mean taking control or re-establishing it in an area of your life, such as with your finances, your fitness, health or your career. Feeling in control is not about controlling other people, but feeling that you are taking responsibility regarding what you want and where you are heading in your life. Control creates confidence and a sense of empowerment.

How well are you 'pulling your own strings' at the moment? On a scale of 1 to 10, if 1 is 'totally out of control' and 10 is 'completely in control', how would you rate the level of control you have in your life? What do you need to do in your current situation to 'get back into the driving seat'?

### Exercise 43: Take action

What do you need to do to feel good about yourself? What do you need to *not do* to feel good about yourself? This will help you to maintain high self-esteem. In simple terms, do more of what works and less of what does not.

### Exercise 44: Give yourself credit

When you look back over your journal you may see some major positive shifts, but because they have taken place over a long period of time, you hardly recognize them. It is important for your self-esteem to acknowledge your growth and development at every step of the way. Use your journal to notice where you have moved forward and celebrate your progress. You may notice, for example, that you have moved from a position of dependence to more equality in a relationship, or from insecurity to self-assurance. Give yourself credit for these shifts and do not allow them to slip by unnoticed.

# The annual review

## Exercise 45: Making an annual review

Stemming from the pillow book (see page 111), you can also keep a brief record of notable events on a monthly basis, from January through to December each year. At the end of each month, note down things you have achieved, any significant experiences or events (good and bad) and any activities you have been part of. You might also want to record the books you have read and the films or exhibitions you went to see, together with your comments.

This would be a good exercise for you if you find it hard to remember the detail about last month or last year, or if you find it difficult to call to mind positive times in your life. It is easy for us to forget the uplifting times and to focus only on the problems. I have done this exercise now for many years, largely because I would otherwise have considerable gaps in my memories, but also because I want to capture what I have done in my life. I know that without my annual review there would be many wonderful moments I would have forgotten and achievements I would have overlooked. A review helps me to remember the richness of my life and reminds me that I have been significant and valuable, thus enhancing my self-esteem.

At the end of the year ask yourself the following questions:

- What was the most fun thing to do?
- What involved the most risk?
- What was the most rewarding thing?
- What was the biggest achievement?
- What was the greatest adventure?
- What involved most friendship and love?
- What was I most affected by?
- What were the biggest disappointments?
- What were my favourite places to visit?
- What was the best new thing?

You might then want to list some goals for the following year.

Using your journal in these ways will help to maximize its benefits for you.

Finally, I wish you well in using your journal to develop the most important relationship you will ever have – the one with yourself.

# Postscript: When the journal is not enough

If you find through working on your journal that overwhelming feelings emerge, please make sure that you take care of yourself and do not try to struggle through alone. This may mean contacting your GP or a counsellor.

The British Association for Counselling and Psychotherapy provides an online list of therapists in all areas of the UK, at www.itsgoodtotalk.org.uk. Telephone: 01455 883300; website: www.bacp.co.uk; email: bacp@bacp.co.uk.

If you are desperate and cannot wait for an appointment, contact the Samaritans (www.samaritans.org), on 08457 909090, where a friendly voice will answer your call 24 hours a day, 365 days a year, or email: jo@samaritans.org.

Alison Waines is a psychotherapist, counsellor and more recently a novelist, writing psychological mysteries and thrillers. Her website is www.awaines.co.uk.

# Suggested reading

Bays, Brandon, *The Journey*, London: Harper Element, 2003.

Bradshaw, John, *Homecoming: Reclaiming and Championing your Inner Child*, London: Piatkus, 1999.

Buzan, Tony and Barry, *The Mind Map Book*, London: BBC Active, 2009.

Cameron, Julia, *The Artist's Way*, Basingstoke: Pan Macmillan, 2011.

Capacchione, Lucia, *The Creative Journal*, Pompton Plains, NJ: New Page Books, 2001.

Dickson, Anne, *A Woman in Your Own Right*, London: Quartet Books Ltd., 1983.

Edwards, Gill, *Living Magically*, London: Piatkus, 2009.

Gawain, Shakti, *Creative Visualisation*, Novato, CA: New World Library, 2002.

Gendlin, Eugene T., *Focusing*, London: Rider, 2003.

Gloubermann, Dina, *Life Choices, Life Changes*, London: Mobius, 2004.

Goldberg, Natalie, *Wild Mind*, London: Rider, 1991.

Hayward, Susan, *A Guide for the Advanced Soul*, Camarillo, CA: DeVorss & Company, 2011.

Huber, Cheri, *There is Nothing Wrong with You*, Mountain View, CA: Keep it Simple Books, 2001.

Jeffers, Susan, *Feel the Fear and Do It Anyway*, London: Vermilion, 2007.

Klauser, Henriette Anne, *Write it Down, Make it Happen*, New York: Simon and Schuster, 2001.

McMurray, Madeline, *Illuminations: The Healing Image*, Berkeley, CA: Wingbow Press, 1990.

Milner, Marion, *A Life of One's Own*, London: Routledge, 2011.

Rainer, Tristine, *The New Diary*, New York: Jeremy P. Tarcher, 1981.

Rogers, Carl, R., *A Way of Being*, Boston: Houghton Mifflin, 1996.

Schneider Myra, and Killnick, John, *Writing for Self-Discovery*, London: Element, 1998.

# Index

121

19658006R00072

Printed in Great Britain
by Amazon